Kate Muir is a Scottish writer and filmmaker. She is the producer of the Channel 4 documentary *Davina McCall: Sex, Myths and the Menopause* and its follow-up *Davina McCall: Sex, Mind and the Menopause*. She is also an activist for The Menopause Charity, dedicated to raising awareness and understanding of the menopause.

EVERYTHING YOU NEED TO KNOW ABOUT THE MENOPAUSE

(but were too afraid to ask)

KATE MUIR

GALLERY BOOKS UK

First published in Great Britain by Gallery Books, an imprint of
Simon & Schuster UK Ltd, 2022

This edition published in Great Britain by Gallery Books, an imprint of
Simon & Schuster UK Ltd, 2023

1 3 5 7 9 10 8 4 2

Simon & Schuster UK Ltd
1st Floor
222 Gray's Inn Road
London WC1X 8HB

www.simonandschuster.co.uk
www.simonandschuster.com.au
www.simonandschuster.co.in

Simon & Schuster Australia, Sydney
Simon & Schuster India, New Delhi

A CIP catalogue record for this book is available from the British Library

Paperback ISBN: 978-1-3985-0566-7
eBook ISBN: 978-1-3985-0565-0

Typeset in Perpetua by M Rules
Printed and Bound in the UK using 100% Renewable Electricity at CPI Group (UK) Ltd

FSC www.fsc.org
MIX
Paper | Supporting responsible forestry
FSC® C171272

For three generations:
Isabella, Ella and Molly

CONTENTS

'And once the storm is over, you won't remember how you made it through, how you managed to survive. You won't even be sure whether the storm is really over. But one thing is certain. When you come out of the storm, you won't be the same person who walked in. That's what this storm's all about.'

Haruki Murakami, *Kafka on the Shore*

I

THE REVOLUTION STARTS HERE

Imagine, for a delirious moment, that men got symptoms of the menopause.

A bloke walks into his doctor's surgery. He starts grumbling:

'My penis is getting all dry and wrinkly. It's agony having sex, but what's the point anyway? My libido just drained away when I hit 50. In fact, I don't know why I bother going to bed. I can't sleep more than an hour with these night sweats, and at work I get so many hot flushes I have to sneak into the gents to change my shirt. Armpits like puddles.

'Have I mentioned the awful anxiety? I wake up before dawn with my pulse racing, feeling like I'm having a heart attack. Suddenly I'm too scared to drive on motorways. I lost the car in Sainsbury's car park. I'm feeling more and more worthless and depressed. Yesterday, I found ice cream melting in my manbag and my phone in the freezer.' He pauses, now tearful. 'Worse still, I'm getting a muffin top.'

Would all this be brushed off as 'men's troubles', reduced to coffee mugs that say 'I'm Still Hot . . . It Just Comes in Flushes

Now!' and largely ignored by the medical establishment? Because that's what happens to 'women's troubles' when many of us are sledgehammered by the menopause and fall apart at home and at work. Ninety per cent of women get symptoms[1] – from hot flushes, memory loss, anxiety, depression and vaginal dryness to fading libido, painful joints and constant insomnia – but they are met with a shrug from society, or a handout of antidepressants from doctors. While not everyone will get the full trolley-load of symptoms, and some will escape with just a couple, the menopause is still woefully misunderstood by many people, including parts of the medical establishment. Women do not need to go through this any more. This is about hope and change, and not the 'Keep Calm and Carry On' attitude that has served women so badly for so long around the menopause. Think of these pages as a capacious handbag of knowledge, stories and cutting-edge science that will help you understand precisely what's happening to your body and mind – and help you to take charge.

This book is part of a newly emerging public conversation surrounding the menopause, through which we can support each other, our colleagues and our partners. Too often, the menopause is still a place of shame. We mention it discreetly as 'The Big M', in the way that a few years ago we used to refer to 'The Big C' of cancer. Even the early feminist menopause books in the '90s euphemistically called it *The Change* (Germaine Greer) and *The Silent Passage* (Gail Sheehy). We need to name, shame, blame and reframe the menopause. It's a subject we barely have the vocabulary for: medically, 'menopause' means the exact day twelve months after your periods stop – it was minted by a Frenchman in 1821 from the

Greek *mēn* (month) and *pausis* (pause). Like most people, I'm using 'menopause' in a wider way to mean that chaotic period of hormonal change that begins with the perimenopause and includes the rest of your life that follows, post-fertility. The older term 'The Grand Climacteric' perhaps describes it better, and I fancy the idea of 'The Reboot' myself, but let's stick with the menopause.

We need to reclaim the M-word for ourselves – in every language. But what if, in some languages, no word for the menopause exists? As Dr Nighat Arif, a campaigning GP from Buckinghamshire who serves a large Pakistani community, told me: 'In Punjabi you might say "no periods", and the word for periods is *kapara* – rags or cloth.' This reminds me of when I worked at *The Times*, where one of the male executives used to refer to female journalists on their periods as 'on the rag'. Now we're all 'off the rag', I suppose. Arif added: 'And there's a rarely used Urdu word, *baanjh*, loosely translated as "dried up", "woman who can't have children". I think I prefer "menopause", which is a much kinder word.' Dr Arif has taken to Instagram Live and even TikTok to reach a wider, younger audience of 150,000 followers with her message in Urdu, with the occasional untranslatable gynaecological word in English cropping up.

The menopause should be about metamorphosis, not misery. This book is about the coming medical revolution that will make most menopause symptoms history and about the parallel need for a cultural – and personal – reboot that celebrates, rather than denigrates, this moment of change. As the menopause movement grows and we reach tipping point, we need to be empowered with up-to-date knowledge of our bodies and our selves.

In the UK and USA, most of us will live for more than 30 years post-menopause, and we'll keep on working for much of that. We need to become much better informed about hormones and safe hormone replacement, and not let the medley of symptoms or the long-term health effects of the menopause bring us down. By 2025, 12 per cent of the world's population will be menopausal – and increasingly vocal. We will be one billion women. Hear us roar!

The sooner we understand everything about the menopause, and its dastardly little sister, the perimenopause, the better we will be primed. This knowledge is not just for older women, but every woman who believes in equality in the second half of life. And keeping a weather eye out in your thirties for the coming storm of the perimenopause in your forties just makes good sense.

We need to start by educating ourselves. I read a shelf-load of books during pregnancy, but in my forties I headed unknowingly into the perimenopause – those pre-menopausal years of rollercoaster hormonal dips and humungous periods that arrive like unpredictable tsunamis. I thought the perimenopause was just the run-up to the menopause, and not a potentially treacherous passage in itself. I had no idea it would make me so furious. In the kitchen at various times during my deranged perimenopausal mood swings, I threw at the wall: 1) a butternut squash 2) *Nigella Christmas* 3) broccoli 4) a full butter dish and 5) blue poster paint. No one was injured. Indeed, the missiles actually released family tension, and at least the dog began to treat me with more respect. Yet despite these clear (if messy) warning signs of growing mental chaos, my full knowledge of the approaching menopause was this: *Periods stop. Full stop. Not a problem. And whatever you do, don't touch hormone replacement therapy.* I was so wrong, I wrote this book.

I'd like to say that this investigation of the failure of the medical establishment and society to manage the menopause came out of my own 'journey', but to be honest my journey was a total car crash. Yet I feel that if so many other women have shared their stories with us for this book, I should, too. At 51, I went off the menopausal cliff in the manner of *Thelma and Louise*. Before then, I had a full-time job as a film critic, three teenage children, a husband, a dog and a mother with late-stage Alzheimer's disease. I lost all of those – some for a short while, some for ever – as we shall see in later chapters. It was not all about biology – psychology, morality and midlife chaos played their part too – but I had absolutely no idea how important hormones were to physical and mental health. As the psychotherapist and writer Susie Orbach put it: 'The menopause arrives, seeking out our vulnerabilities like a guided missile, just as we need all our strength to cope with daily life.'[2]

I thought I was capable of coping with anything until I met the perimenopause and menopause. I thought I was in control. But my passage through midlife's magnificent shitshow has been an education that has both put me in my place and helped me understand how tough that place is for others. At the same time, I don't underestimate the liberty bestowed by the end of fertility and child-rearing, and how much of a relief the menopause must have been in the past, and still is for some women today, particularly the lucky ones who romp cheerfully through 'The Change'. Freedom – not just of speech – and late-life leadership and creativity are glorious gifts. In the nineteenth century, the US suffragist and abolitionist Elizabeth Cady Stanton argued, after having six children, that women could move from domestic concerns to wider ones as they aged. Stanton 'believed that menopause had redirected all her "vital forces" from her reproductive organs to her brain.'[3] She and her fellow feminist Susan B. Anthony toured America, speaking at rallies and having racy adventures of all sorts. As one observer wrote, 'stately Mrs. Stanton has secured much immunity by a comfortable look of motherliness.'[4]

Ageism and the über-visual values of the Instagram, TikTok and selfie age keep the menopause festering in the closet. While in Ye Olde England there's also still the charming legacy of crones, witch-burning and glycolic facial peels, many cultures, particularly African and Asian, have far greater respect for older women and the wise words of the 'auntie', or the elder. The 'grandmother hypothesis' is huge in anthropology: in *The Slow Moon Climbs: The Science, History, and Meaning of Menopause*, historian Susan Mattern[5] sifts our primaeval past and suggests that the menopause helped our success as a species. In hunter-gatherer tribes, grandmothers, who could provide childcare and extra food supplies while consuming little themselves, were incredibly useful to the community. But because women's lives were so short, menopausal grandmothers were rare creatures.

Now, as we live into our eighties on average, grandmothers are about to be huge. In *Flash Count Diary: Menopause and the Vindication of Natural Life*, author Darcey Steinke studies a community of killer whales, or orcas, one of the few mammals that has a menopause like us.[6] Recalling the background to her book, she said, 'I was struggling and needed my own totem to move me through menopause. There're some amazing older women, but a lot of them are sort of continuing to keep their façade of their fertile life intact and so when I found the whales and I found that they go on to lead their pods after they go through menopause, I realized nobody offers them hormones. Nobody tells them that their vagina is dry. They just become badass leaders. It really inspired me.'[7] Steinke discovered that pods are most successful when led by grandmothers, who run the show and know where to find the best salmon. She kayaked in the sea off Seattle, waiting for the whales to breach: 'The wild matriarchs have given me hope,'[8] she says in the book, impressed that the 'granny' whales were neither frail nor apprehensive, but in every way leaders of their communities. 'They demonstrate to me what no human woman could: that it is not menopause itself that is the problem but menopause as it's experienced under the patriarchy.'[9]

Yet so many who are going through the menopause fail to rally or lead because they are crushed by debilitating symptoms and loss of confidence. The transition is made worse if they are already facing discrimination or disability. Nine out of ten women in the UK experience menopausal symptoms but most of them get no support whatsoever. A 2022 Channel 4/Fawcett Society survey showed 14 per cent of women in the UK use hormone replacement therapy (HRT).[10] In the USA, three quarters of menopausal women who ask for medical help are left untreated[11] – and that's the lucky ones, who are insured.

Once you look at life through the lens of the menopause

and its silent, often devastating effect on mental health and women's confidence, many mysteries are explained. The peak time for female suicide is between the ages of 45 and 49, the typical years of the perimenopause, and the attrition continues into the early fifties. The focus on the public drama (and indeed comedy) of hot flushes as *the* sign of the menopause, coupled with mass ignorance about the perimenopause, means many women blame themselves, rather than their mercurial hormones, when life falls apart. Yet by the time symptoms such as hot flushes are manifesting, the hormone decline has been going on for as much as a decade. Hormones start sporadically draining away in women's forties, and some find changes starting in their late thirties. One in 100 women experience menopause under 40, a huge, mostly invisible demographic. The end of periods occurs on average around 51, but five years either side of that is perfectly normal too. Hormones are anarchic. If only I'd known that the perimenopause was in many ways a second wine-soaked puberty, and if only I had talked about it back then with my friends, I'd have created far less chaos for myself and my family.

While female health concerns, particularly for women past fertility, are dismissed as trifling by society, this is worsened by an *omertà* among women themselves. The previous generation completely failed to tell us what they went through, and they knew very little anyway. I had just one – unforgettable – conversation with my mother, Ella Muir, about the menopause. In her forties and fifties she worked as a personnel manager in Stirling Glen's, a dusty, old-fashioned department store on Argyle Street in Glasgow. Her office had fluorescent lights and partition windows onto a dingy corridor where everyone went by. She grew tomato plants on her windowsill overlooking the street. One day she came home, shocked, and told me: 'My period suddenly started and it was so heavy my chair was completely covered in blood. I had to call the girls in from the office next door to bring a towel. They taped sheets of newspaper up on all the windows so no one could see in, and we cleaned it up. Awful, just awful. I was so embarrassed.' That was her last period, all she ever said about the menopause to me, and to my shame, I never asked for more. I was 13 then, and my own, brand-new periods were of much more interest.

Yet I remember after the menopause, Ella became obsessed with her thyroid gland, even though the doctor repeatedly said it was fine, and she sometimes complained of being under the weather, although her normal mode was high-heeled, whip-smart and bustling, as in retirement she volunteered at the Clydebank Citizens Advice Bureau. Occasionally she went mysteriously ruddy-faced. My mother couldn't find any reason for her strange symptoms and feelings. After her death, when I cleaned out her flat, I found a folder of yellowing newspaper cuttings on thyroid disorders, obsessively annotated in increasingly wobbly writing. I guess thyroid problems might have been what she mistakenly blamed for her menopausal symptoms and the brain fog that eventually became Alzheimer's disease.

Unlike my mother's generation, we are the generation that will fight the menopause revolution, supporting and empowering each other on social media and in life. But are we so much better at communication? Although I'd been researching this subject for nearly two years and producing and writing the Channel 4 documentary *Davina McCall: Sex, Myths and the Menopause*, when I asked my daughter, now aged 21, to read my script synopsis, she came back and said: 'Great, but what's the perimenopause? You should explain that.' Like most of her contemporaries, she uses an app such as Clue to track her periods and moods. Menopause apps are just coming into circulation now, so I hope with femtech and more openness, my daughter will be a great deal more prepared than her mother or grandmother. She'll know that the perimenopause brings an unpredictable mixed bag of symptoms that can encompass anything from fatigue and mood swings to heart palpitations, anxiety and migraines, and often women blame those on the normal stress of forty-something life when in fact hormonal imbalance is the culprit. Tracking symptoms on a free, medically accurate app like Balance Menopause Support really helps women to get a picture of their own health. For many women, one clear physical sign of the perimenopause is changes in their periods – mine became unpredictable deluges, but many others' just dwindle away. Detailed medical studies of perimenopause symptoms are seriously lacking – perhaps because there is no obvious start to The Change, unlike the ending of periods that occurs in the menopause – and that needs to be addressed, although one recent Swiss study showed that lower estrogen levels were mirrored by increased depression in the perimenopause.[12]

Indeed, many of the symptoms of the perimenopause are the same as in the menopause itself: when you scroll through the Balance app now, there's an epic, almost gothic list of about 50 symptoms – from bloating, memory loss and tinnitus to vaginal dryness, migraine, hair loss and even 'irritable legs' – and useful suggestions for how to ease them. Lots of menopause books have mysteriously plumped for 34 symptoms, and the Greene Climacteric Scale, a tick-box list used by many researchers and doctors, has 21. When scientists ask menopausal women about their symptoms, 80 per cent report hot flushes,[13] 77 per cent report joint pain,[14] and 60 per cent memory issues.[15] Aside from these three, further plagues of the menopause include: heart palpitations, sleeplessness, anxiety, depression, headaches, panic attacks, exhaustion, irritability, muscle pain, night sweats, loss of libido, vaginal dryness, body odour, brittle nails, dry mouth, digestive problems, gum disease, dry skin, hair loss, poor concentration, weight gain, dizzy spells, stress incontinence – and last but not least, something that might be from a horror movie: formication, which means an itchy feeling under the skin, like ants. I had that. Quite simply, the majority of women battle through the menopause, and only a lucky few are symptom-free.

Obviously, unless you're super-unlucky, you only get a few of these symptoms, and knowing your enemy really helps. Where would we be without Dr Katharina Dalton, the British scientist who identified the hormonal dip of premenstrual syndrome, or PMS, in 1953,[16] at last giving women the tools to understand their monthly mood swings? (Where is Dr Dalton's Nobel Prize for services to women? At least we can nominate her for a blue plaque at London's University College Hospital in 2024, twenty years after her death.) Being alert to PMS allowed women to cope better and feel supported. We need to have a similar shout-out for the hormonal swings, roundabout and helter-skelter of the perimenopause and menopause, and if women are largely ignorant of this, most men know diddly-squat. We need to bring them on board. When I told some gentlemen-of-a-certain-age that I was writing this book and making a documentary on the subject, they looked simultaneously horrified and embarrassed, like I'd been drunkenly sick on their shoes. Fertility signals worth: a new 'trophy wife' tends to have functioning ovaries, and the word 'menopause' has a whiff of witchiness. But there were other men who listened intently, had stories about their wives and partners, and wanted to understand better this new, angry, sleepless creature that was sharing their bedroom, hot in a whole new way.

'Knowledge is power, especially when it comes to health.'[17] So says former First Lady Michelle Obama, who has used hormone replacement therapy ever since a hot flush floored her on the presidential helicopter. She gives graphic details of that burning epiphany in her podcast. 'I'm dressed, I need to get out, walk into an event, and literally it was like somebody put a furnace in my core and turned it on high, and then everything started melting. I thought, "Well, this is crazy. I can't, I can't, I can't do this."' Menopause in high places, from helicopters to the West Wing, could have had a seriously detrimental effect on world politics, but fortunately Michelle Obama got medical help and President Barack Obama got on board too. 'Barack was surrounded by women in his cabinet, many going through menopause, and he could see it, he could see it in somebody, because sweat would start pouring,' says Michelle. 'And he's like, "Well, what's going on?" And it's like, "No, this is just how we live," you know? He didn't fall apart because he found out there were several women in his staff that were going through menopause. It was just sort of like, "Oh, well, turn the air conditioner on."' It's so important that men, employers and colleagues get educated and share the burden, so it is no longer carried by menopausal women alone.

This is an uplifting example of fitting one's working life around the menopause, but millions of women have less understanding bosses than the former president of the United States. It's carnage out there in the workplace, but you can't hear anyone scream. One in ten female workers leaves their job because of menopausal symptoms,[18] a shocking statistic. Another survey showed nine out of ten women felt symptoms negatively affected their performance at work[19] and many quietly dial down to part-time roles. All that wisdom, expertise and maturity is being needlessly chucked away at huge cost, in roles ranging from highly qualified nurses to powerful executives. There is a hormonal layer on the glass ceiling. In Chapter 4, we'll look at ways to smash that.

Even if we are shameless about the menopause, and talk about Menopause Power as loudly as the younger generation talks about Period Power, we still face a fatberg of fake news and sloppy science in our understanding of this huge hormonal transition. Medical research has focused so long on the average male that the average female has been atrociously neglected, as Caroline Criado Perez shows in her radical investigation *Invisible Women: Exposing Data Bias in a World Designed for Men*.[20] The book exposes the gender data gap at the root of systemic discrimination against women, and this medical sexism is also at the heart of the scandalous neglect of the menopause.

How many people know what actually happens in the menopause – to half the planet's population? At around the age of 51 – or younger, in more deprived communities – periods stop and the triumvirate of super-powered female hormones – estrogen, testosterone and progesterone – disappears. After up to a decade of hormonal decline, women are left high and dry. The menopause is not just a transition, but the start of a hormonal deficiency that risks having a negative impact on a woman's future health, in the form of osteoporosis, heart disease and dementia. It's worth taking these risks seriously, even if you are one of the lucky ones and have an easy, graceful transition with few or no symptoms. For everyone, the menopause marks a health watershed that merits attention in terms of lifestyle changes. And if you are interested in your healthspan, and not just your lifespan, then hormone replacement therapy is worth looking into. Historically it has had a bad rap due to a misleading and highly damaging report that came out in 2002, which we will be discussing later in the book, but safe and effective HRT is now readily available, and we will come to the best HRT choices in Chapter 8.

What actually goes on during this transition is astonishing. So much is the opposite of what you'd expect. For instance, which hormone do women produce more of: estrogen or testosterone? The answer is testosterone, which most people consider to be a male hormone. We just produce less than men, but testosterone is hugely important for female sexual pleasure, energy and mental health – yet it is not officially prescribed 'on licence' for women on the NHS drugs formulary list as part of HRT, even though it is an essential hormone that should be replaced, according to menopause experts.[21] It's a still a struggle to get testosterone 'off licence' – i.e. as a special dispensation using a small amount of the gel which is licensed for men – from your GP, even if you confess your libido is dead as a dodo and your brain is misfiring. It's a perfect example of medical sexism. Is there some resistance, perchance, to females over 50 being sexy and smart? Men with low levels are given replacement testosterone for libido on the NHS, but not women. Men can buy Viagra over the counter for £19.99, but there's no equivalent for women. Why is male midlife sexual pleasure prioritised over female?

This explains why so many women in their fifties throw in the towel in bed and pick up a garden trowel instead. Over half of women say the menopause has negatively affected their sex life.[22] Some find happiness in hobbies. I'm an avid vegetable gardener, but I want more than that. Women accept the menopause as their wretched lot, another silent burden to bear after the end of pregnancy and periods. They are resigned to low-level misery, medicating with prosecco and paracetamol. Respect to those who can ride out into the hormonal desert without help, but I wasn't one of them. Eventually, when prosecco failed me, I decided to try replacing my missing estrogen, progesterone and testosterone.

HRT vanquished all my symptoms and, although for many women the changes take weeks or even months, astonishingly it started to bring me back from the brink within just four days. My hot flushes disappeared forever and my brain clicked back into gear. I stopped throwing household objects and began reading scientific papers. I have been taking HRT for six years, and if possible I intend to stay on it forever. I now use what the best menopause specialists recommend – body-identical hormones derived from yams. In my case this is transdermal (through the skin) estrogen which I apply as a rub-on gel twice a day although it is also available as patches, and a micronised progesterone pill at night, both available on the NHS. I had to get my testosterone cream privately for years – but after three attempts I recently got it on the NHS.

Once I had sorted my own hormonal basket case, I wanted to find out more about HRT and other medical options for women, as well as conducting an open-minded (and occasionally hilarious) investigation into alternative treatment options for those who cannot or don't want to take hormones (see Chapter 7). Tackling the menopause is holistic work. But sometimes a healthy lifestyle and a kick-ass attitude is just not enough. I had a two-year, health-endangering struggle to get the safest HRT (more of which later), and the more I discovered the shocking lack of care and information for women, the angrier I got. I interviewed extraordinary doctors and exceptional women who had fought for their own health. If, as a white, middle-class, straight, cis reporter, I had been dangerously messed around and couldn't find out the truth about the safest treatment, how hard was it for women with less time and fewer resources? I changed from patient to journalist to activist in the space of a year. The more I found out about what happens to women going through the menopause – physically, mentally, medically and culturally – the more I went to war.

The cavalier dismissal of the menopause reflects a wider injustice in healthcare and hormone therapy. For trans men and some non-binary and intersex people – depending on hormone use and whether and when ovaries and womb are removed – the menopause can be emotionally triggering, as well as a physical struggle, and this is discussed in Chapter 6. Although I use the term 'woman' in this book for simplicity, I also want be inclusive of people in menopause of all genders who were assigned female at birth, and who are on different hormonal journeys. London psychotherapist and counsellor Tania Glyde (they/she) started the website Queermenopause.com, a very useful resource, and has recently published research on the LGBTQIA+ menopause experience and the need for better education of therapists and doctors.[23] Increasingly, the movement is telling its own menopause stories.

The Covid-19 coronavirus shone a klieg light on science's and society's failure to pay attention to differences in health outcomes depending on ethnicity, class and sex, as the pandemic hit Black and Asian communities much harder. So far, white women tend to be the public face of the menopause movement, but Black women often have the hardest time, with the menopause starting earlier, at 49 on average, and hot flushes remaining a symptom for around ten years,[24] compared with six for white women. Meanwhile, women from South Asian backgrounds in the UK are much more likely to get postmenopausal osteoporosis. More specific research needs to be done, and more diverse menopause stories need to be told.

Karen Arthur began her @menopausewhilstblack feed on Instagram in those stressful months in 2020 after the first Covid-19 lockdown and during the growth of the Black Lives Matter movement following the murder of George Floyd. Arthur was a London teacher but became a fashion designer as she rebooted her life during the menopause. She also launched a survey of the menopause experiences of Black Caribbean and Black African women based in the UK. 'When I googled "menopause", I scrolled down and all I saw was images of sad-faced, white-haired white women," she told me. "You'd think that Black women didn't get the menopause.'

With her robust, confident attitude to the menopause, which

we can all learn from, Arthur is changing all that. She decided to start navigating the transition with therapy, mindful meditation and healthier eating. Her brilliant YouTube[25] video on overcoming depression during the menopause has her swapping colourful outfits as she chats, until suddenly she's confidently down to her navy bra and pants. 'Falling in love with my little pot belly has meant that I'm much, much better . . . When I do open my mouth, what I say is valid and important. Wearing clothes that lift your mood is not dressing for men or dressing for women. It's dressing specifically for you. Wear what you fucking like, when you fucking like it! If you are willing to grow and learn about yourself during menopause, then that gateway to your next phase of your life is liberating.'

Arthur fills me with hope whenever she talks about the menopause, but you have to be determined enough or lucky enough to reach that gateway, which is not always possible for those with life-shattering symptoms. Menopause can also be eased with time and enough money: vitamins, bespoke nutritional programmes, aerobic exercise, yoga, therapy, essential oils and retreats. But if you work full-time in the gig economy or live with poverty, obesity or a disability, menopause care is often hard to access or non-existent. For many, self-care is an expensive, time-consuming luxury, not a necessity. Discussing – never mind complaining about – menopause in a difficult family or workplace situation is a risk many women dare not take. The divide between those who have menopause support and knowledge and those left to suffer is massive.

In particular, the divide between the Have-HRTs and the Have-Not-HRTs is shameful; the rich get their hormones privately and often secretly, sometimes with a touch of Botox and filler, while the poor struggle to get any help at all. Some old-fashioned NHS GPs still refuse to prescribe HRT altogether,[26] and it is women who are already struggling with compromised health that need it most. As Dr Kate Pickering, a GP on the frontline in Glasgow for three decades, explained to me: 'If you're ten floors up in council flat in Easterhouse and you're a grandmother getting up to look after a baby because the mother is looking after the other kids and you've got night sweats – well, HRT should be bog standard to help. Menopause is a big issue, and there's not enough information available. No one ever talks about working-class women and it's a real inequality.'

We need to talk about the menopause everywhere, and with social media the conversation is getting louder and stroppier. The feminist columnist Caitlin Moran recently went viral when she compared the perimenopausal crash to 'coming off Ecstasy' and suggested you are better prepared for the comedown if you took a lot of drugs in your youth.[27] Hormones, she said, 'make you feel a bit stoned and lovely'; while we still have estrogen flowing, we are 'high on nature's sexy Valium . . . kinder, gentler, more self-sacrificing'. Afterwards, we take revenge. There was also a high-five response on Instagram and Twitter when Kristin Scott Thomas gave her classic menopause speech in Phoebe Waller-Bridge's television series *Fleabag*. 'Women are born with pain built in,' said Scott Thomas's glamorous, sharp-witted executive character. 'It's our physical destiny: period pains, sore boobs, childbirth – you know. We carry it within ourselves throughout our lives. Men don't . . . We have pain on a cycle for years and years and years, and then, just when you feel you are making peace with it all, what happens? The menopause comes, the fucking menopause comes, and it is the most wonderful fucking thing in the world. And yes, your entire pelvic floor crumbles and you get fucking hot and no one cares, but then, you're free, no longer a slave, no longer a machine with parts. You're just a person.'

Actually, the good news is that you can now be a person *and* have a non-crumbly pelvic floor post-menopause, but your doctor probably hasn't mentioned that. You do not need to suffer vaginal dryness, a shrivelling clitoris, recurrent urinary tract infections and a lost sex life if you use topical estrogen regularly on your vulva.[28] A little estrogen cream or a pessary can make a huge difference. Considering the effort and expense we dedicate to erasing wrinkles on our faces, you might think we would give our vulvas similar attention. It would be life-changing if every GP asked every woman in midlife about her undercarriage.

The outpouring of relief and personal stories that came after Davina McCall's menopause documentary in May 2021 astonished me. Social media erupted as #davinamenopause trended on Twitter, every newspaper carried features and there were follow-up radio phone-ins where women shared their survival techniques – and their often-unnecessary suffering. McCall was startlingly honest in the programme, explaining how she was told *not* to talk about the menopause at work as it was somehow 'a bit unsavoury', and discussing her symptoms, from brain fog when trying to read autocues to a dry vagina and sweats that made her ask 'Is this make-up chair heated?' She was no longer the presenter of *Big Brother*, but the nation's 'Big Sister', said one newspaper, giving the menopause taboo the kicking it deserved. 'I have never had a reaction to any TV programme quite like it,' McCall says. '*Big Brother* was big, but after we made the menopause documentary, people were literally stopping me everywhere I went to tell me their stories. I was on social media every night with other menopause warriors, just trying to help women.'

The film had over one million viewers on broadcast, and one million more on catch-up a few days later as women told their friends about the show. GPs reported women coming in saying: 'I'll have what Davina's having,' after McCall put on an estrogen HRT patch on camera, and Sally Harris, a pharmacist in Wales, tweeted: 'I dispensed more HRT yesterday than I'd normally do in a month!'[29] In the year after the programme, NHS HRT prescriptions rose by an unprecedented 42 per cent, according to the Nuffield Trust.[30] I'm an activist for The Menopause Charity, which was set up by doctors and campaigners, and we launched just two days after the documentary aired, offering one free professional, six-hour, online Confidence in the Menopause course to every GP practice. Over 11,000 GP surgeries in the UK signed up in the first two months – a sign of how keen doctors and nurse practitioners are to provide better care. If every one of those new-found menopause experts treats 100 patients, over 1 million women across the UK will have been given better menopause care.

That thirst for missing knowledge is an indictment of the state of NHS menopause care, and evidence of how little it matters to those at the top of the medical bureaucracy. GPs and even obstetricians and gynaecologists are not to blame – education is the culprit, as is the ten-minute consultation. Although the menopause will happen to every woman in the world, and has massive health consequences, according to a Menopause Support investigation, 41 per cent of UK medical schools do not give mandatory menopause education.[31] Dr Rebecca Gibbs, an ob-gyn consultant at the Royal Free Hospital in London, told me: 'When I trained at Barts ob-gyn, it was 2003–4 and nobody took HRT because you were going to "die from cancer". At medical school I went to possibly one lecture on it, tied into things like puberty. That was it.' A Mumsnet poll in 2020 showed that 36 per cent of perimenopausal women and 26 per cent of menopausal women who sought help for their symptoms visited their GP three or more times before being offered appropriate medication or help, and a third said their doctor told them they'd just have to 'learn to live with it'.[32]

For all the fancy talk in the medical establishment of 'person-centred pathways' and 'patient choice', there are few options if your practitioner is not informed. Dr Madeleine Lameris is a menopause specialist and a GP tutor at Cambridge University who is working on a new student curriculum. She says, 'Women are hitting brick walls quite a lot in menopause. It's dangerous if GPs are not educated, because the risks are higher in the really old HRT preparations. Better menopause education should be a mandatory part of the RCGP [Royal College of General Practitioners] curriculum.' You have to be a detective to find 'menopause' in the GPs' core curriculum.[33] At the moment, it gets a mention under 'Gynaecology and Breast', in a section titled 'Other'. Lameris explains that GPs can update their knowledge with extra, fee-paying courses, but many just muddle along – 'and they can be very defensive if women come in with information and they don't know about it.' The British Menopause Society (BMS) offers professional training courses, with a £400 weekend introductory course followed by half-day training shadowing a menopause specialist over three to six months (which can either be free or cost up to a few thousand pounds, depending on the generosity of the hospital or practice), but I recently met a doctor who had waited three years to be allocated her training placement. Post-pandemic, the BMS has plans to put more courses online, which should help.

Right now, however, if doctors are not informing women, then women must inform themselves. The time has come for feminism to catch up with science, and for science to catch up with feminism. Germaine Greer's opinions are now outdated and controversial in many areas, but her embrace of the 'natural' menopause as an escape from the male gaze has a certain liberating oomph: 'If a woman never lets herself go, how will she ever know how far she might have got? If she never takes off her high-heeled shoes, how will she know how far she could walk or how fast she could run?'[34] Yet at the time Greer wrote this, in 1991, medical studies of the menopause were even more limited than they are now. Now that we are aware of the scientific research, maybe we can take off our high heels, but also take advice from the intersectional feminist Audre Lorde: 'Caring for myself is not self-indulgence, it is self-preservation, and that is an act of political warfare.'[35]

It's going to be a long war. In Victorian times, we flushed warmly off to heaven by the average age of 59, barely giving the menopause time to matter. We were done and dusted, delighted that childbearing was over. Now, one in four women in the UK will have a 100-year lifespan,[36] with half of that time hormone-deficient, and as the long-term effects of this deficiency become increasingly understood, it's evident that this puts them at huge risk.

Long lives are not always easy ones: my mother died at 89 of Alzheimer's, horribly aware, for a time, of her mental decline. Watching a parent slowly disappear into the smog of dementia is a peculiar agony. I'm a daughter of Alzheimer's. I have a 22-year-old daughter, and the risk travels down the female line. Along with dementia, Alzheimer's is the biggest cause of death for women in the UK. So, what excited me most in researching this book was the cutting-edge science on the protective effect of estrogen on the brain. Replacing estrogen in a 'window of opportunity' around the start of the menopause reduces the chances of dementia and Alzheimer's.[37] We need to encourage more research and get that news out to a wider audience.

This isn't just a guidebook. This is a manual for revolution. The menopause need not be a test of silent suffering. We can eradicate or significantly lessen most menopause symptoms – and just talking about them openly can be a source of instant relief. The menopause is one of the few areas of medicine where healing can be easy, and protecting long-term health is an added bonus. In the words of British menopause specialist Dr Louise Newson, who runs the largest menopause clinic in the world, was one of the inspirations for this book, and set up The Menopause Charity to empower women and educate doctors: 'Our vision is to make menopause symptoms a thing of the past, something that's only read about in history books.'

Whether we follow Karen Arthur's idea of a 'gateway', or the Japanese word for this phase of life, *konenki,* which translates to 'renewal years' and 'energy', or the Chinese *dì èr gè chūntiān,* 'second spring', there needs to be a massive cultural shift on this subject. The silence around the menopause needs to become a cacophony, and, one day, a symphony.

2

NOT WAVING BUT DROWNING

There is a famous poem by Stevie Smith, 'Not Waving but Drowning', which has almost become a cliché. Yet it kept coming back to me when I was thinking about the chaos and madness that the perimenopause brings by stealth upon women. Smith wrote the poem when she was 55, about onlookers who ignore a man dying at sea, his frantic panic mistaken for cheerful waving. The man writes from the afterlife:

> 'I was much further out than you thought
> Not waving but drowning.'[1]

I realised that as hormones unpredictably drain and refill like rip tides in the perimenopausal years, when women are usually in their forties, it is not merely the onlookers, families and friends that don't realise what's going on. We ourselves have no idea. We still have our periods. We still think we are waving, when in fact we're drowning.

For me, the perimenopause was the elephant in the powder

room. I still had my periods when I got a few hot flushes in my late forties, and when I told my GP she said, 'Oh, you're too young to be menopausal. They can't be hot flushes.' I was in her surgery because I'd started getting lots of erratic heart palpitations in the night: sudden, fast, panicky pounding in my chest and tightness in my throat, for no reason at all. She sent me for an electrocardiogram, at some expense to the NHS. I'm a runner. My heart was fine. The doctor's diagnosis was 'too much coffee'.

Of course, now that I've read umpteen menopause manuals and academic papers, I know that those harmless palpitations were a classic and common sign of falling estrogen levels, and reported by more than 41 per cent of perimenopausal women.[2] My doctor, however, did not. Nor did she seem know – thanks to the gaps in GPs' training – that hot flushes and night sweats are reported by 10 per cent of perimenopausal women.[3] The perimenopause should have its name up there in throbbing red warning lights, because its shifty symptoms so often get mixed up with the regular stresses of forty-something or (more rarely) late thirty-something life, particularly for women holding down a job and holding up a family.

The effects of the perimenopause on mental health are powerful, and barely acknowledged. The anxiety, mood swings, sleeplessness, flat depression and irritation are bad enough, but outbreaks of rampant perimenopausal rage – particularly if you've been a calm, chilled person previously – are a sign that loving, gentle hormones are no longer holding back the real, raw you. Add that to the hormones roiling in your teenage children, and it's an evil brew. A bestselling novelist and menopausal ice-water swimmer that I know remembers 'the rage' well: 'My teenage daughter was arguing with me across the kitchen and I thought, *I'm so angry I'm actually going to kill her.* I really wanted to. Infanticide – just a bit late.' And then the insanity passed.

The hormonal fluctuations of the perimenopause are like the weather: measure them on one day and you'll find estrogen and progesterone are up, but on another they'll be in the doldrums. This is why those over-the-counter pinprick blood tests for menopause sold by pharmacies are often a waste of money, never mind inaccurate. You send off a drop of blood in a vial to a private testing centre and receive a breakdown of your hormone levels, but only for the day you drew the blood – as Dr Louise Newson says, 'You can have low estrogen at 3 a.m. and get night sweats, but be back to normal levels in the morning.' Such tests do, however, include leaflets that warn that the results are hard to interpret and not always reliable in the perimenopause.[4] The tests measure your levels of follicle-stimulating hormone (FSH), which for normally menstruating women rises every month to stimulate the growth of egg follicles. If the level is much higher than normal, usually over 30IU/L, you're heading into the perimenopause and menopause as the body struggles to pump out its last eggs; post-menopause levels can be 70-90IU/L. For women who think they might be in early menopause, a proper blood test from your GP is more useful, but it's not usually necessary if you're at a typically menopausal age. Quite simply, your symptoms tell the story. 'The NHS wastes millions every year on largely unnecessary tests for women over forty-five,' says Dr Newson. 'If symptoms like hot flushes appear, you know your estrogen is low and you can consider HRT, even if you still have periods.'

Some people barely notice the perimenopause at all, while for many it creeps in slowly. Medical guidelines often suggest the average duration is four years, but science is lacking on that, and more research needs to be done. Some women find perimenopause lasts up to ten years. But you already knew, from years of periods, that hormones are diabolically unpredictable. The physical symptoms of the perimenopause can include: sleeplessness; sore, swollen, lumpy breasts; migraines and headaches; exhaustion; weight gain; and food intolerance and bloating – all of which are easily conflated with the usual hormonal ups and downs of periods. Other symptoms of perimenopause are similar to the menopause itself, with vaginal dryness, brain fog, fatigue, hot flushes and night sweats rolling in as hormones and periods peter out. Another clue is that your cycle may get shorter or longer in the perimenopause. In addition, as the advice leaflets say mildly, 'You may also get heavier periods.' In my own case, this was a ridiculous understatement compared with the graphic gushing and terrifying clot-flushing that occurred. I only dared go to work when heavily armed with Super Plus Tampax – in pairs. Obviously, I told no one. But it turns out that these colossal periods affect 44 per cent of perimenopausal women.[5]

Though I didn't realise it at the time, I was running on empty. I was still having periods at 51, along with tropical flushes. My nights were damp and feverish, but I ignored that, along with the gathering loss of sleep. I woke most mornings before dawn in panic and tears, feeling like a limb had been amputated. I was also in the throes of divorce, which brings its own insanity and guilt. My two sons were abroad and at university, but my then 15-year-old daughter was left in the maelstrom of a dying marriage, and I felt I'd utterly failed her. I busily pretended to myself and those around me that this was not happening at all, physically or mentally. I just kept on running. I went to work every day as *The Times'* chief film critic, tried to look after my daughter, attended film festivals across the world, from Cannes to Toronto, campaigned for equality with Women and Hollywood, interviewed directors and actors live on stage, did broadcast interviews and recorded *The Times Film Show* video every week for the newspaper's website. Being on camera or on stage always brought on a humdinger of a hot flush, and I sometimes sneaked into the toilet to change into an identical black top for continuity. No one noticed – apart from me.

If fluctuating estrogen was sending erratic electrical signals to my heart and internal thermostat, what peculiar messages might it have been sending to my mind? Your brain and every part of your body, from your joints to your vagina, is filled with estrogen receptors. In the perimenopause, unless you're one of the lucky women whose body cruises through the process as smoothly and smugly as a Tesla, there is a feeling of being puppeted by forces outside your control. Hormones play good cop, bad cop: soothing you one minute, abandoning you the next, depriving you of sleep and breaking you down. When the nurturing hormones estrogen and progesterone start disappearing, that often leaves testosterone dominant, till it goes, too.

'As your perimenopause gathers pace, you experience what I can only describe as increasing sobriety,' Caitlin Moran, who is 45, wrote in *The Times*.[6] 'Suddenly the poor behaviour of other adults comes into focus, as you deal with your hormonal hangover. You don't have any "lady forgiveness" left in your tank.' Instead there's growing anger: 'You want to meet up with your coven of similarly menopausal friends, all of you stoking each other's fires of outrage.'

You can often cope with anger for a while, relieving it as I did by throwing the occasional vegetable across the kitchen. But sometimes the build-up of frustration goes beyond that. Most women have spent a couple of decades putting their kids, ageing parents, employers and sometimes partners first, and the self that emerges after the caring mummy-hormones begin to disappear can be liberating as well as terrifying. It was for me. People talk about mothers – never fathers – juggling work and home, but it's less juggling and more suppression of the woman's needs. Her needs to be nurtured, to have space, and, above all, time. Suddenly a little mercurial perimenopausal voice inside says: 'Go on, just drop the juggling balls!'

Skye Gyngell, the Michelin-starred chef who opened the Petersham Nurseries restaurant in London, dropped all her balls (and knives) at once. 'I went through a really difficult period between 45 and 48. I felt like I was completely unravelling and unwinding and I couldn't work out what was happening to me,' she recounted in an interview on the inspiring MPowered Women menopause website.[7] 'I left the house that I'd lived in for 15 years, the man that I'd been with and had a young child with, the job that I loved and had made my name at. I literally jumped off the precipice without wings.' When I read that interview, I felt a humungous sense of relief. *You too*, I thought. Why did no one talk about this perimenopausal kamikaze instinct? I called up Gyngell to hear more. We talked for an hour. She told me: 'I didn't know about the emotional effects of perimenopause. I just thought I was living my life on the hamster wheel, between school runs and the restaurant, and I was neglecting my relationship and completely exhausted and disgruntled and couldn't work out why. A forty-hour week isn't possible in a restaurant – everybody works a sixty-hour week or more on their feet. Sometimes I used to have to go to bed and sleep for twenty-four hours. I literally hit a wall. And then I threw the baby out with the bathwater . . .' Of her precipitate escape, she added: 'It was menopause insanity, but I only see that in retrospect.' She has now rebounded with a new restaurant, Spring at London's Somerset House.

Hearing that made me feel so much better. I was completely unequipped for my own implosion in 2015, after my mum died of Alzheimer's disease. Things had already been going wrong, and I had an affair with a married man. A few months after my mum's funeral, I left my husband, my home, my three kids – one of whom was still in school. Suddenly I found I was living by myself in a rented flat, drunkenly building an IKEA Malm chest of drawers at midnight, waking up in an anxious sweat before dawn, desperate to see my daughter, who was away for much of the week, and deeply ashamed of the collateral damage and pain I had caused. But I could breathe again. Obviously, all of that cannot be blamed on cold turkey when hormones disappear. My responsibility is clear, including a long marriage we should have looked after with more care. But it took the perimenopause to disable the brakes and propel me into that *Thelma and Louise* moment.

The nexus of the midlife crisis and the hormonal crisis is a dark theatre, where many apparently happy couples act out parts that were written years ago and need updating. Jane Haberlin, a London psychoanalytic psychotherapist who works with individuals and couples, and also coaches professional women, often deals with this midlife combination in her patients. She finds that the perimenopause is literally and figuratively a wake-up call. 'What seems common is so many women are awake in the middle of the night, at 3 a.m. or 4 a.m., when any worries are magnified. They're disturbed, not sleeping, lying next to someone they're perhaps no longer having sex with, or in a relationship where there's no kindness.' Often men are equally discombobulated – or bored – staring into another half-century of monogamy as our lives grow longer. I'll talk more about relationships in Chapter 12.

The struggle to cope with the hot mess of the menopause, accompanied by the loss of the protective buffer of hormones, can bring up serious trauma repressed for years, which may require professional counselling. Even if this isn't the case, for most of us this is a time of questioning, breaking-down and rebuilding. Haberlin thinks the Generation X cohort coming into the menopause now has very different, and higher, expectations of relationships to those preceding. 'Our mothers' generation were often deeply unhappy and bitter, felt trapped. I wonder how many of them had a terrible menopause that they never spoke about, how many were on Valium?'

Those of us who may now live to 100, and work until 70 at least, find ourselves pushing the boundaries in our work and home lives. Haberlin explains: 'You can question whether you've been made unhappy enough that you have the courage to make a break. You have another 30 years and is this how you want to live your life? Some people worry about things like pensions, cling to a marriage that might be very much over, and rationalise their unhappiness away. Others leave, have a panic attack, ask, "What have I done? I've made myself insecure."'

In early menopause and divorce I had a couple of whopping panic attacks on the cliff-edge of insecurity. Once, I found myself staying at a friend's house in Wales, missing my children who were away elsewhere on holiday, and I woke up alone at 4 a.m. unable to breathe, gasping, crying, heart battering my chest. (The only time I'd ever experienced this before was in a plane that tried to land three times in a lightning storm at Glasgow airport.) The feeling was of pure terror and a need to flee. I got in my rental car (with my newish puppy, Skye, in the back) and drove erratically into the dawn, shaking. It was only when I found myself falling asleep at the wheel on the M4 that I realised how unstable and dangerous I was. I stopped in a service station. Skye had a pee, and then we slept together across the back seat for an hour. The experience brought me to my senses and made me go and talk to a therapist. But that insecurity, that panic at every new day, does not last for ever. And panic sometimes makes you take action. As Skye Gyngell told me: 'When one door closes, another one opens. It's just the corridor between them that's scary.'

One of the forces pushing at the door is sexual desire, thanks to the ovaries and adrenal glands still producing some testosterone. As calming progesterone falls, testosterone and erratic surges of estrogen may become dominant. In Chapter 12 I discuss the phenomenon of the perimenopausal 'sex surge', which happens to some women. Temporary testosterone dominance perhaps makes us more determined to get what we want at work and in bed. As journalist Christa D'Souza suggests in her menopause book *The Hot Topic*, testosterone is the hormone of infidelity, estrogen is the hormone of compliance. 'I couldn't bear the idea of going to my deathbed never having slept with anyone other than my husband ever again,' she says. 'To be really honest, I couldn't bear the idea of sleeping with my husband again.'[8] Hormone treatment helped D'Souza. While some women feel the urge to throw in the tea towel and run from long-term relationships into the arms of someone else, temporarily or permanently, others find their sex drive dies away with their diminishing hormones, leaving a perilous imbalance in a relationship where a man is still raring to go (or on the testosterone or Viagra that the NHS prescribes for men but not women, who have an equal need). For lesbian couples, the menopause can sometimes be an out-of-sync double whammy – or a time of mutual support.

The hormonal hell of the perimenopause and menopause can be far more dangerous than a break-up. Suicide is at its highest for women aged 45–49, and at its second highest in the 50–54 age group. (There are similar midlife peaks for male suicide.) Female thoughts of suicide seem to mirror hormonal fluctuations, as well as menopausal depression, which is different from clinical depression. Menopausal depression usually responds to hormone treatment, but less so to antidepressants. Therapy is not always the answer, either. Patients who have never previously been depressed describe low mood – 'a grey, flat kind of feeling, a loss of joy', says Dr Rebecca Lewis, a former anaesthetist and GP turned menopause specialist, who has a particular interest in menopausal mental health. Lewis consults with dozens of menopausal women every week at the

Newson Heath Menopause & Wellbeing Centre in Stratford-upon-Avon, and says: 'The reason women come to see me most in the clinic is not the hot flushes, not the muscle pains, but the psychological changes. As eggs begin to run out in the perimenopause, that starts fluctuations in hormones which affect the brain's limbic system, which governs anxiety, mood, libido and concentration.'

Estrogen is a neurotransmitter, docking to the outer membrane of neurons in the brain and passing on signals. Think of it as your hormonal Wi-Fi connection. The amygdala, the part of the brain that processes emotion, is packed with estrogen and progesterone receptors, so when hormones dip, so does mood. Low estrogen is to blame for premenstrual syndrome and post-natal depression, as well as menopausal depression. Anxiety can be overwhelming at the best of multi-tasking times for midlife women, but add emotional-hormonal loss to that and there's serious risk. Lewis points out that women in their forties and fifties are also part of the wilting-sandwich generation, handling both ageing parents and antsy teenagers. They expect to have it tough, just not this tough.

Women are also scared to admit to what is often called 'menopausal brain fog' – forgetting words, names and appointments. Around 73 per cent of perimenopausal and menopausal women struggle with brain fog,[9] as hormones disappear from the hippocampus, the region of the brain concerned with memory. This can leave you halfway through a sentence . . . with no idea why you began, as transmitters fail in your brain. The fog also seems to cause household objects to move in mysterious ways. As television presenter Davina McCall – who I worked with on the menopause documentary – told me:

'My phone was in the fridge and my keys were in the bin. I had trouble concentrating on the autocue – colleagues were asking me what was wrong. I kept going and I didn't tell anyone. I was ashamed.' Women fear the scrambled brain is a sign of early dementia. It's probably not, and most seem to get over the mild deficits by training the ever-plastic brain to make new connections. But if you have a challenging, competitive professional life, losing even a tiny bit of cognitive capacity may be hard to take, particularly when the *Daily Mail* unhelpfully refers to the memory loss as 'pink fog'.[10] That nagging, silent fear adds to the depression.

Karen Arthur, who started @menopausewhilstblack, suffered anxiety and depression as her hormones bailed out. I interviewed her a few months after the first Covid-19 lockdown in London, and she pointed out things were even tougher for Black menopausal women then, isolated at home while videos of racist killings by police were showing on a loop – 'And that's on top of the trauma that's been going on for ever.' Her own menopausal breakdown – or breakthrough, as she prefers to call it – came when she was still a teacher, with two grown daughters. She was sitting in a school meeting, feeling anxious about the amount of work she still had to do, when the fire alarm went off. Rather than assemble for the fire drill in the usual way, she gathered all her things and just walked out. 'Something went inside me. I finished my work for the day at home, and I thought if I go to bed now the morning will come quicker. I burst into tears and called my friend, who advised me to go to my GP.' The doctor signed Arthur off work for a week, and then months. 'I was screening phone calls, eating really badly, creeping out to the nearest shop, hiding from anyone who knew me. I realised the hot flushes were not because my boiler was broken! I'd thought that I needed to ring British Gas.'

She went away for a restorative seaside weekend – and found herself, aged 52, walking to the top of Beachy Head, the infamous suicide spot. 'Those thoughts that had come into my head lying under the duvet returned, thinking it would be lots easier for everyone if I wasn't here. But standing on top of a cliff, I realised very clearly: that's not what I want to do. I want to be here.' The doctor told Arthur she was depressed, 'But I thought, *That's what happens to other people.*' She was offered anti-depressants but declined, preferring to first try a more holistic approach to recovery. She went into therapy for three years and says, 'That's the best gift I've ever given myself. The menopause forced me to be honest with myself and the people around me. I'd spent a decade not being me and it was exhausting.'

I went the same route, trying therapy for the first time ever for about 18 months in early menopause. Being Scottish and repressed Presbyterian by background, I had of course considered psychotherapy to be weakness and self-indulgence, but I was, once again, wrong. My therapist was very practical and feminist. She basically handed me the emotional toolkit that I'd been raised without. She made me look at the rusting scaffolding beneath my relationships, pointed out to me that no one can guess what you are thinking unless you tell them, and explained that avoiding conflict was possibly a bad idea. In summary, the 'Keep Calm and Carry On' mantra that so many of us resort to in midlife needed an emergency overhaul. I started looking after myself, mopping up the mess I'd made for others and reconnecting with my children. And I agree with Arthur about the honesty: it's time to tell the truth.

If you can afford therapy, midlife is fertile territory, with so many key changes happening in terms of relationships, empty nests, dying parents and work-life balance. Perhaps the shorter, cheaper route of some midlife coaching will be enough, or just walking and talking with best friends, which has stood me in good stead for the past five years. Unfortunately, therapy is almost impossible to get quickly on the NHS, particularly for the amorphous muddle of the menopause, and a lot of women just end up walking out with antidepressants after a ten-minute visit to a doctor. Indeed, in one study of around 3,000 British menopausal women, after complaining of the onset of low mood or anxiety, 66 per cent were offered antidepressants by their doctor instead of hormones.[11] During the Covid-19 pandemic, prescriptions of antidepressants were at an all-time high.[12] They offer an easy solution. Valium was nicknamed 'Mother's little helper' in a 1966 Rolling Stones song, and now modern equivalents like Prozac, Seroxat and Cipramil are seen as 'Granny's little helper' instead.

It turns out that the use of antidepressants is embedded in the medical system. Through the Quality Outcomes Framework, GPs' practices are paid bonuses per patient – incentives for diagnosing all manner of illnesses like depression, diabetes, high blood pressure and asthma, as well as encouraging contraception and discouraging obesity. But, as I was shocked to learn, they are paid nothing extra for diagnosing the menopause and perimenopause, or for prescribing HRT. That's not a 'quality outcome', apparently. There is effectively a financial disincentive: your GP gets paid better for diagnosing depression than they do the menopause.

I spoke to Dr Zoe Hodson, who was a GP in Manchester before becoming a menopause specialist. 'Doctors are not driven by this. That's not what we think about when we see a patient,' she said. 'We don't need to bash GPs, but what we do need to address is changing the Quality Outcomes Framework to include menopause. You can't always properly help a menopausal woman in a ten-minute consultation. Sometimes you need a double appointment, and that's not easy to justify to the financial manager in the practice.'

In a piece of NHS doublethink, the government's National Institute for Health and Care Excellence (NICE) says in its guidelines that HRT should be the *first choice* when it comes to medically treating menopausal psychological symptoms, and that 'there is no clear evidence' that antidepressants ease low mood in menopausal women.[13] 'I come across a lot of women who are given antidepressants as first line and HRT is not even discussed,' says Dr Louise Newson. 'But the treatment does not often work because it is a different set of causes . . . there are hormonal reasons for having these symptoms. But antidepressants can be useful for hot flushes for some people, particularly those who choose not to take HRT, although they are often limited by their side effects.' These side effects can range from drowsiness to dizziness, and antidepressants can often destroy what's left of your faltering libido – SSRI antidepressants are infamously known as 'orgasm blockers'.

In the UK, 16 per cent of women in the 45–64 age group take antidepressants.[14] In a survey of prescriptions in America, an astounding 20 per cent of women in their forties and fifties took antidepressants, and that rose to 24 per cent in women over 60.[15] That figure is from 2018 and has probably grown post-pandemic. Something is going badly awry if almost a quarter of women are on antidepressants in the years post-menopause. A need is not being met.

Dr Michael Craig, a consultant psychiatrist who set up the innovative Female Hormone Clinic at the Maudsley Hospital in London, told me the connection between depression and lack of estrogen has been proven again and again, 'but somehow it falls between two disciplines, gynaecology and psychiatry. GPs could fill that holistic void and look at the whole person.' But GPs don't, because they have no time in those ten-minute consultations, when patients are supposed to raise only one item.

Craig points to a double-blind randomized controlled trial where perimenopausal and early postmenopausal women were given HRT containing transdermal estrogen and micronised progesterone.[16] Only 17 per cent of those on HRT developed any depressive symptoms, compared with 32 per cent on the placebo. Using this HRT halved women's chances of low mood. 'Estrogen affects neurotransmitters and serotonin. We see that in all forms of reproductive depression,' says Craig. 'Women who get PMS [premenstrual syndrome] and postnatal depression tend to be the same ones who suffer problems during the menopause.'

If only Craig's and others' work on treating perimenopausal and menopausal depression with HRT had been better known a decade ago, the life of Janice Wilson, a 52-year-old former nursery teacher from Yorkshire, might have taken quite a different turn. I heard about what had happened to Wilson when I first went to Dr Louise Newson's clinic to get my own HRT sorted out, and what began as a personal consultation became political. It made me so shocked and so angry, it became the catalyst for researching this book. At the age of 43, Wilson went to her GP with a whole list of typical perimenopausal symptoms, none of which her doctor recognised – and Wilson ended up being given twelve sessions of electroconvulsive therapy (ECT) in a mental hospital instead.

Wilson agreed to talk to me, although for family reasons, we have changed her name. She said she had always struggled with her hormones for two weeks out of every month, suffering with the low mood and anxiety of premenstrual dysphoric disorder (PMDD), and had also experienced post-natal depression. But those clues to hormonal imbalance were ignored by Wilson's doctor. 'My internal thermostat wasn't working – I was either too hot or too cold. I still had my periods, but I was perimenopausal. The first symptoms were urinary, then depression and anxiety – it hit me like a ton of bricks. The anxiety wasn't about an event or a particular reason. Just this terrifying anxiety. I'd wake every twenty minutes or so during the night with a bad dream.'

Like many undiagnosed perimenopausal women, Wilson was sent on an odyssey of NHS specialists with her various symptoms. (In one survey, almost 20 per cent of women had five or more hospital appointments and investigations before hormone problems were diagnosed.[17]) 'I went with symptoms to a neurologist, a urologist, a gynaecologist and various GPs, but the hormone question was always brushed aside. I'm a shy, quiet person, so I found it hard to make the point. I was never offered a blood test to check my hormones.' Instead Wilson was fobbed off with antidepressants. Then a locum psychiatrist diagnosed her as bipolar in a 30-minute consultation and she never saw him again. 'That stayed on my record, and no one thought to look beyond it. The antidepressants just left me flat, and when each antidepressant failed to work, they found another and another, with their own side effects.'

A year after trying all these anti-depressants, Wilson was diagnosed with 'treatment-resistant depression', and ended up having ECT as an outpatient. Each time, she was given a general anaesthetic before electrode pads were placed on either side of her head and 180–460 volts of electricity were fired through her brain. 'I can remember the first treatment and some of the second but very little after that. The building was very foreboding and I was terrified they would lock me up. I had to get onto a bed surrounded by people and equipment. That was hard, as I'd become very afraid of medics. Afterwards my jaw was quite painful – I imagine that was caused by the muscle contractions. I was befuddled, unable to organise my thoughts to have a conversation. That time is such a blur.'

The blur lasted seven years, as Wilson withdrew from the world and had severe memory loss. 'I couldn't feel love for my children or husband; in fact, I felt very little, other than fear that often became terror. At those times, I would be desperate to tear my skin off and escape the body that I felt didn't belong to me. I sat in a chair with the curtains closed all day. I sat in silence, didn't answer the phone or see any of my friends. When my husband came home, I'd put on the telly so I looked like I was doing something.'

Eventually, she attempted suicide. 'One night I took much more medication than I should have. It wasn't a cry for help. I just needed it to stop. Waking up that morning was absolutely devastating.'

But the shock of surviving focused her mind enough to start an internet search, and she read about reproductive depression being treated with transdermal estrogen. Wilson also discovered that women with similar symptoms to hers were being treated with HRT at a private menopause practice, then in Birmingham, run by Dr Newson. She decided to make an appointment.

But how would Wilson get there? She was anxious and agoraphobic. She couldn't even bear to go to the shops or walk her dog. How would she travel so far with the severe urinary tract problems she was suffering? At that point, Wilson and her husband had a mad eureka moment. 'We took out an extra mortgage and bought a camper van, drove down there, and parked it outside the clinic.' Wilson felt safe in their mobile home-from-home, and got up the courage to walk in the clinic door by herself. After that, everything fell into place. Newson prescribed HRT: estrogen patches, progesterone, and a testosterone cream specially for women.

Wilson was astonished by the speed of the change: 'My depression was gone within days. Days! It was just miraculous. I started sleeping straight away, and the anxiety that was with me constantly just lifted.' And something previously impossible happened: 'I went out into the garden with my dog.'

Now completely off her antidepressants, Wilson takes HRT and uses topical estrogen to help with urinary problems caused by dryness around her vulva. She is living a full life again, reunited with her family and friends. Her mental-health team were astonished, agreeing she had never been bipolar – and a few of them went for specialist menopause training, following her case. One even started HRT herself.

The use of electroshock therapy is an extreme example, but the consistent misuse of antidepressants and the under-use of HRT is a scandal that is causing not merely misery for women, but huge, unnecessary costs for the health service. The instant verdict of female depression has grim echoes of Victorian physicians diagnosing menstrual and menopausal symptoms as 'hysteria' and getting out the leeches, straitjackets or ice baths. The word *hysteria* derives from the Ancient Greek, meaning 'wandering womb', which was believed to cause all sorts of female trouble. 'It is altogether erratic,' wrote the Greek physician Aretaeus of the womb, back in the second century AD. Millennia of patriarchal thinking needs to be overturned here, and plenty of books have already been written on the centuries of othering of women and their mysterious, occult hormones. We know that 13 of the 16 women accused in the Salem witch trials were of menopausal age,[18] and 'climacteric insanity' i.e. menopausal madness was a popular reason for committing Victorian women to asylums. Sigmund Freud referred to menopausal women as 'quarrelsome, vexatious and overbearing'. Actually, I think it's time we were quarrelsome, vexatious and overbearing about the menopause, or nothing will change for the better.

As Karen Arthur said, 'the menopause gave me a voice', and we need to speak up about mental health in midlife, so that we can move forward. When Arthur came out the other side of therapy, she became a fashion designer and sewing tutor, and at 60 she is an advocate of making conscious clothing choices to lift your mood (#WearYourHappy). I visited her studio complex in Catford, south-east London, where she works alongside dozens of other artists. Her own space is a wild cornucopia filled with gold lamé, second-hand silk scarves, African textiles and skirts upcycled from printed coffee-bean bags. The other presence is the energy of Arthur herself, who was cutting out and pinning patterns as she talked to me, a pink, lime-green, gold and orange mural forming a backdrop behind her. 'Pockets are a feminist issue,' she pointed out, and said she always includes them if she can.

Arthur's Instagram is as colourful as it is political, and now she is using it to specifically survey Black menopausal women in the UK: 'because our stories seem to have been ignored amongst this vast landscape. I'm not an expert on menopause but I am expert on, and vocal about, my own experience and I am committed to having more women who look like me sharing theirs and giving hope to others.'

Arthur is still navigating some symptoms, from aching joints to itching legs, and has made numerous changes to her lifestyle to combat this, including changing her diet to include more fruit and vegetables, and less alcohol. 'I eat more healthily, but I like chocolate and a tot of rum sends my hot flushes through the roof. I realised menopause isn't a transition to be gotten through; it's something to live within.' Arthur worked on tweaking her routine and she curated her life to help with her postmenopausal needs and ambitions. Whether you are on HRT or not, 'The Change' requires some life changes, and for me, for Arthur and for Gyngell, it unexpectedly marked not just a turning point, but a whole new life and purpose.

It's easier to understand what has happened in retrospect. As Skye Gyngell explained to me: 'All the crazy things I did with menopausal insanity were really good in the long run. I'm happy with the outcome now, but I would have chosen to do it a different way.' At 58, she has more energy and clarity than she did a decade ago, and believes she never would have been brave enough to leave the restaurant and her relationship without her hormonal crash. Looking back on the wild years of transition she said: 'You can't swerve it. I think you have to be proactive and think, this is what it is, nothing's going to change that, so how can I do it mindfully and with enough information and enough strength to go into it confidently and challenge it – challenge the perceptions of what the menopause is?'

I agree. Now that I'm at the other side of hormonal and emotional chaos, I'm happy hanging out with my grown-up children and I have a new partner, new work, some new friends as well as my old ones, a new dog and a new set of hard-earned tools for dealing with life. Gyngell has already done a huge amount with her life in recent years, and told me she plans to do much more: 'Technically I should retire in seven years, but I feel I've got twenty more years of work in me, more to offer now the dust has settled.'

We all have different menopauses, and different needs. We just need to talk openly about that, and support each other through the hormonal maelstrom. Gyngell added: 'There is a way to get through. Remember that children's book *We're Going on a Bear Hunt*? I loved that book. Every obstacle he came across he said, "We can't go over it, we can't go under it, we've got to go through it." It's an amazing little life-lesson that book. *You've just got to go through it*.'

3

HORMONES

The Holy Trinity – Estrogen, Progesterone and Testosterone

Why do women know almost nothing about the smorgasbord of symptoms served up by the perimenopause and the menopause? Why do we blame ourselves for everything that goes wrong? Why do we remain so ignorant of the saturnine hormones controlling our moods, our relationships, our orgasms, our energy, our pregnancies, our periods and our menopause? Hormones are the car women drive around in every day, yet we've no idea how the combustion engine works. (I like a motor metaphor. My dad was an engineer in a car factory in Glasgow before they were all shut down.) If we paused to consider how estrogen oils our minds and our bodies, from our vaginas to our vocal cords – hence the faltering voice of old age – we might actually service that car and find ways to top up the fuel when it runs out. Knowing how your machine works matters.

Six years ago, I could not have named the three major female hormones – estrogen, progesterone and testosterone – and told you what they did. I knew I'd produced a lot of estrogen when I was pregnant and that falling progesterone levels had something to do with PMS, but I just would not have included testosterone in that set of feminine hormones. Once I lost all those hormones, however, over an erratic couple of years, I realized just how much they mattered.

I don't want anyone to be as ignorant as I was of the coming mental and physical commotion or the extraordinary protective effects of hormones. The menopause is a stage of life, not an illness, but forewarned is forearmed. So let us now take a grand tour of our hormones, and learn of their powers for good, combatting decrepitude and serious illness. It will be a game-changer.

Estrogen

Estrogen is basically the superpower in the female body and brain, and when it disappears during the menopause, its absence causes chaos. Most women keep quiet and soldier on, considering these changes just to be part of the normal process of ageing. They are – but it's the suddenness of the change that shocks. Estrogen leaves women's bodies when they're in their early fifties, on average, but men's testosterone – the lack of which has similar ageing effects – doesn't reach an equivalent low until they're in their eighties. The sudden drop in estrogen explains why women aged 45–55 rush out to spend more than any other group on anti-wrinkle products,[1] as collagen in the skin decreases by 10 per cent over a period of roughly five years when the menopause hits – unless you take HRT.[2] The estrogen crash is also why we suffer more and earlier osteoporosis and dementia than men.

There are three kinds of estrogen: the powerful estradiol, and its weaker sisters estriol (made in pregnancy) and estrone. While you continue to make a tiny bit of estrone even after menopause, in your fat tissue and adrenal glands, and you can give your body a tiny boost with soy products, by the time the ovaries pack up and the estradiol tank empties, you may need bigger guns. I did. In Chapter 8, I go into the science on how much safer the new plant-based, body-identical hormone replacement therapy is, and how starting it in perimenopause and taking it for the rest of your life might be the best option for most women. Body-identical means it's an exact molecular copy of your own estrogen and progesterone. But, in the meantime, bear with me while we celebrate estrogen, not just for its ability to send menopause symptoms packing, but for its powerful long-term protective effects.

'We no longer believe that estrogens are just sex hormones, but important therapeutic targets for preventing diseases as disparate as osteoporosis, heart disease, and neurodegeneration,'[3] said the authors of an article in *Trends in Molecular Medicine* that examined a stonking 162 scientific papers on estrogen. Name the disease, and replacement estrogen – taken through the skin – is here to help, reducing the risk of stroke and heart disease by 50 per cent,[4] reducing the prevalence of colon cancer[5] and helping to prevent type-2 diabetes and high blood pressure.[6] Basically, estrogen works on the cells that line the arteries, keeping blood flow stable and keeping the arteries from constricting. It also eliminates the joint-pain of fibromyalgia and helps with arthritis. The book *Estrogen Matters*, by breast cancer surgeon Dr Avrum Bluming and psychologist

Carol Tavris, is well worth reading and makes a compelling case for replacement estrogen.[7]

Once you start looking at the world through estrogen-shaped spectacles, all sorts of diseases loom into focus. It's revealing just to consider your own family's medical history. What about my mother's cataracts? (A tricky combination with Alzheimer's disease, to say the least, but the doctors did manage to remove one.) What about my aunt Grace's blurred vision due to macular degeneration? With two out of three cases of blindness affecting women, was hers caused by the strain of a long career in teaching, or a lack of estrogen? Does estrogen provide protection against blindness, as well as lessening the day-to-day discomfort of dry eyes? Why, yes, it does. The lens of the eye is covered in estrogen receptors, and it turns out that starting HRT around the onset of menopause reduces the occurrence of cataracts and lowers the chances of macular degeneration.[8]

What about my grandmother, Isabella McCusker, who had multiple sclerosis? I barely knew her before she died, still dark-haired in her sixties, but I remember that when I was a toddler she would generously put up with me bouncing on her and bonking her on the head with a Johnson's Baby Powder bottle as she lay every day, unable to walk, in the bed-recess in her tenement kitchen in the village of Old Kilpatrick near Glasgow. Estrogen is not a treatment in itself for multiple sclerosis, but three studies of multiple sclerosis patients who used HRT[9] reported an improvement in their symptoms – one by 75 per cent – and a better physical quality of life. Doctors also noticed that when MS patients were pregnant, the high natural estrogen levels at that time had a remarkable therapeutic effect and reduced relapses. A growing body of research shows that replacement estrogen can lower inflammation as well as making relapses less frequent.[10] What if we'd known that when my grandmother was alive? Would we have needed to cram the wheelchair, the tartan rug and the daft spaniel in the boot of the car every holiday, or would Isabella have been more able to walk?

Perhaps the most important effect of estrogen for most women is keeping their bones strong. Half of women over 50 will have an osteoporosis-related fracture, compared with one in five men,[11] but most have no idea until the break happens that their bone density has lowered. The dangers are insidiously invisible. My friend Louisa Young, an author and songwriter, recently discovered she had osteoporosis when she broke her arm in six places. She has written 11 novels and collaborated with her daughter Isabel Adomakoh Young on the Zizou Corder *Lionboy* children's series. Young is therefore the ideal person to put into words what it's like to suddenly find, after the menopause, that your bones have turned to porcelain. 'I think of myself as a sturdy, strong person, not a skinny, bent-over little Polish countess with brittle bones. But it turned out I had a skeleton made of glass,' she told me. Previously, Young went everywhere on a Harley-Davidson motorcycle, and dressed the part. 'I had no symptoms, I was well nourished, and then I broke my humerus [upper arm bone] tripping over the doorstep. It's one of the biggest, strongest bones in your body. You'd maybe expect to get six breaks crashing a motorbike into a wall, but just tripping over?'

Somehow, I'd always imagined bones to be solid, made from some sort of human marble, but they are more like the trunk and branches of trees and constantly renew themselves. Professor David Reid, a consultant rheumatologist and osteoporosis specialist, explained: 'Bones turn over all the time. A small piece of bone will renew in three to nine months. That renewal becomes a problem because estrogen is very protective to bone, and when it fails in menopause, the forming of the new bone can't keep up with the breakdown of the old.' He compares a frail, osteoporotic bone to an Aero bar: 'lots of holes and not much chocolate'. A healthy bone is more like a Wispa inside.

Professor Reid recommends weight-bearing, high-impact exercise like running, tennis or dancing, with their constant jolts to the skeleton, to help increase bone-mass density when it declines due to estrogen starvation after the menopause.[12] How steep is that decline? 'Two or three per cent of bone mass is lost every year, from just before menopause until a woman is about sixty. Then it slows down a bit, to about one per cent.'

So, for the average woman that's a 20 per cent bone-density loss over the decade after periods stop. (Osteopenia or low bone density usually entails a 10 to 20 per cent loss, and osteoporosis is over a 25 per cent loss.) Bone loss is less if you work very hard indeed to maintain density through exercise, a calcium-rich diet or take a vitamin D3 supplement which also helps bones absorb calcium. While postmenopausal bone loss is already a risk, chronic heavy drinking makes it much worse.[13] However, the good news is that moderate alcohol consumption – say, a glass of wine a day – may help maintain bone density.[14]

American studies show that white or Asian women get osteoporosis at twice the rate of Black women,[15] and being thin and petite makes it more likely you will develop the disease. Dr Nighat Arif campaigns to bring menopause information to Pakistani and Indian communities in the UK: 'We find women who have covered up all their lives here have a severe deficiency of vitamin D – which helps the body absorb calcium – and they'll not mention any menopause symptoms at all until suddenly they'll be hanging up the washing and fall over and break a hip.' Osteoporosis is politely nicknamed 'the silent disease' but it's actually a stealth bomber, with no symptoms at all until a tiny strain, bump or fall smashes bones.

Bones weakened by osteoporosis often shatter into pieces, rather than cleanly crack. Young's arm was too badly broken to operate on at the time, so she was given a brace. 'They hoped the bones weren't too displaced and they'd heal themselves naturally.' She slept upright for four months to keep the bones aligned. I remember her Instagram back then showed a sunlit breakfast in bed, crisp white sheets, and a pile of promising novels. The reality was grimmer. 'It was massively debilitating for a year, and I couldn't drive. There was no comfortable position to sit or write in, and I was up to here with painkillers. Eventually the knob of bone at the top reattached itself, but they had to operate on the rest. I've fourteen screws and a huge piece of titanium in my arm. They gave me good drugs and a great scar.'

After the break, Young was diagnosed with osteoporosis and had a DEXA scan, a low-level body X-ray that shows up bone density. 'It turned out my bones were weakest at the base of my spine. I'm fucking lucky I found out before I ended up paralysed.' She was then given zoledronic acid – 'injected in a chemo chair for half an hour' – once a year for three years.

The drug slows down bone breakdown, increases bone density and decreases the amount of calcium shed from the bones into the blood. 'I'm a nice hippy in many ways, but I wasn't going to reject a bit of modern medicine. Manuka honey and a little light Pilates isn't going to cut it.'

The break happened a week after Young's sixtieth birthday, at which point she had never particularly considered the risks of osteoporosis. She had coped with the menopause transition without help during her early fifties, at a time when she was under huge stress looking after her terminally ill fiancé, 'so I suppose the menopause didn't bother me. Proportionally it wasn't comparable, and it wasn't going to kill me'. (Her devastating, resilient memoir, *You Left Early: A True Story of Love and Alcohol*,[16] is Young's account of that relationship.)

Some women don't even know they've had a fracture, as Professor Reid sometimes discovers when he sees a woman's DEXA bone scan: 'I'll ask a patient, "Was it painful when you got that fracture in your spine?" and she'll say, "What fracture?"' And we all know what a series of small spinal fractures does, leaving older women stooped, caricatured as the ancient, witchy crone of fairy tales. This makes me wonder about my own mother, Ella, who was a strapping 5ft 1ins on her passport but only 4ft 11ins by the time she died, and that was without an osteoporosis diagnosis. She always wore sturdy little heels to compensate.

So, what should women, particularly those with a family history of osteoporosis, do? The most commonly used drugs for slowing bone loss are called bisphosphonates – usually alendronic acid, zoledronic acid or denosumab. Bisphosphonates decelerate the breakdown of bone, letting the bone-building cells work more effectively. There is also a promising new drug, romosozumab, that builds bones and reduces the risk of fractures. At time of writing it has not been approved by the NHS except in Scotland, but it is available privately for a whopping £9,000 a year. With many of these drugs, there is a small risk of osteonecrosis, when cells in the jawbone start to die, and treatment should be paused. Another downside is that these drugs are mostly used only following a first fracture – after the skeleton horse has bolted.

So, why not prevent osteoporosis with estrogen supplementation rather than treat it at huge expense afterwards? The British Menopause Society says that estrogen 'remains the treatment of choice for osteoporosis prevention in menopausal women, and especially in those with premature ovarian insufficiency [early menopause]' and that 'HRT reduces the risk of both spine and hip as well as other osteoporotic fractures.'[17] Could Young instead start using transdermal HRT to rebuild her bones, even after 60? Professor Reid says Young's bisphosphonates 'could be combined with HRT if someone was keen to try, and had a friendly gynaecologist'. Doctors are increasingly looking into the 'slow drip' start of estrogen in small amounts for older women, which gently opens up estrogen receptors that have been shut down for years.

Yet still the medical establishment as a whole remains mysteriously blind to estrogen's superpowers, stuck in its separate silos of cardiology, endocrinology, rheumatology, ophthalmology and gynaecology, unable to see the big picture. 'If you're not even looking at the 55-year-old woman in front of you as being menopausal, then you're missing a whole part of who she is,' says Dr Stephanie Faubion, medical director for the North American Menopause Society.[18] 'Until doctors see menopause as a threat to health in general, they're not going to take it seriously. They're going to say, "This is one of those female things that will go away."'

The 'one-size-fits-men' approach has been challenged on a global scale by the Covid-19 pandemic, in terms of gender and ethnicity. As we now know, white women with Covid-19 have much better survival rates than Black, Asian and some other ethnic groups, who are hit disproportionately harder, and two thirds of all Covid-19 deaths are male.[19] Interestingly, while obesity and other 'underlying conditions' increased rates of death, estrogen seems to decrease them – research has shown that younger women who typically have higher levels of estrogen in their bodies were more likely to survive and more likely to have milder symptoms from Covid-19. Estrogen (and testosterone) supplementation also seems to help some women suffering from Long Covid.[20]

Female Covid-19 mortality rates suddenly start to increase as women hit their fifties, after the menopause.[21] Estrogen enhances the immune system in women, while testosterone has an immunosuppressive effect on men. Covid-19 is clearly a sexist infection, but after over a year of worldwide carnage, research has barely started to understand the ways in which it affects male and female differently (and those of different ethnicities). There is a gender data gap here that is not just irritating, but life-threatening. Should men have received the vaccination first? Interestingly, a study published in 2021 looking at over 5,000 Covid-19 cases in women showed that women who were using any form of HRT were 78 per cent less likely to die of Covid-19.[22] Would topping up the estrogen in women who needed it have made a difference?

This protection can be explained because estrogen regulates immunity and inflammation,[23] which may be why that terrifying 'cytokine storm', which rips Covid-19 patients apart in hospitals, is less severe in women than men. Why did the medical establishment not prick up its ears early on when a study from Wuhan in China showed that women with low estrogen levels had worse infections?

Following that Wuhan report, other promising news about female immunity started to appear. The British ZOE Covid Symptom Study app showed that women taking the combined contraceptive pill (combining estrogen and progesterone) seemed to be less likely to catch Covid and less likely to end up in hospital if infected.[24] Later, a TriNetX global database survey of 17 countries showed that women taking estrogen HRT were 50 per cent less likely to die of the virus.[25] The pill and HRT seemed to offer some protection. But such useful news got much less publicity than, say, former US president Donald Trump shouting about hydroxychloroquine or bleach as Covid cures.

The early signs are promising, but more research is needed – studies following the trail from hospital to patients at home with Long Covid. An online survey of 1,294 women suffering the miserable symptoms of Long Covid found the majority reported that their periods had changed and said their symptoms were worse before or during their periods, when estrogen levels are at their lowest.[26] Covid affects the ovaries, too. It turns out the virus is not merely vicious, but prone to hormonal mood swings.

Long Covid is particularly prevalent in women over 50, and aside from respiratory problems, the reported symptoms have a huge crossover with those of the menopause – insomnia, brain fog, joint pain and heart palpitations. Dr Louise Newson says: 'These symptoms are likely to be related to low estrogen and low testosterone levels, so consideration should be given, as a priority, to replacing these low hormone levels with the right dose and type of HRT.' Newson and others have treated a number of Long Covid patients of menopausal age with HRT, including estrogen and testosterone, and their Long Covid symptoms have improved. But, so far, there's no mention of hormonal help on the Long Covid section of the NHS website,[27] and no large-scale academic studies have been done on this specific area. Other relevant research has been fast-forwarded in these times of trouble, so why have female hormones been left behind?

Just why have estrogen's superpowers received so little attention? I'm reminded of when I started work as a film critic, over a decade ago, and none of the superhero blockbuster movies then starred any women. Female critics started asking why we had Batman, Spider-Man, Iron Man, X-Men and Ant-Man but at that time not a single woman holding her own in the multiplexes. Then, as pressure and interest grew, Wonder Woman, Captain Marvel and Black Widow arrived, to a strong box office response. Let's think of estrogen as Wonder Woman's magic force-field bracelets, and give it the attention it deserves.

Progesterone

Progesterone is a key player in our bodies. The hormone boosts energy, helps sleep and soothes mood, nourishes hair and skin, lightens periods and encourages bone-building cells. Its role in thinning the lining of the womb also helps protect against uterine cancer, by countering estrogen's stimulating effect on the tissues of the uterus. When progesterone is good, it's very, very good – but when it's bad, it's horrid (to paraphrase the poem).[28] When progesterone and estrogen levels fall, just before a period, that's the downer that leads to premenstrual syndrome, or just general malaise and grumpiness, for a few days. But for an estimated 5 per cent of women with an increased sensitivity to progesterone, there can be a much more serious negative mood-reaction – premenstrual dysphoric disorder (PMDD) which can last for one to two weeks. Women who have a tendency to PMS or PMDD often have a harder time in the menopause, as we saw with Janice Wilson, in Chapter 2, who was given electroshock therapy when her hormonal problems were wrongly diagnosed. As a last resort, some women with PMDD opt for a hysterectomy and removal of their ovaries, taking estrogen alone afterwards. Some women with progesterone intolerance cannot take oral HRT – although sometimes taking progesterone vaginally in pessaries or a coil works instead.[29]

When it comes to HRT, progesterone is a key player, and we'll discuss this further in Chapter 8. Understanding that progesterone comes in two very different forms in HRT – natural progesterone or the synthetic progestin – may change the future for millions of women and their doctors. (The spellings are irritatingly similar. Childishly, but usefully, I always remember natural progesterone has 'one' in it, and is one of us. Progestin has 'in' in it, and is a foreign *in*vader. It's also sometimes spelled progestogen.) Progesterone is found in our bodies, rising in the second half of the monthly cycle, after ovulation, while 'micronised progesterone', made from yams, is a structurally identical copy of the hormone – 'micronised' just means it is in tiny particles, which are easier to absorb. Body-identical micronised progesterone is what's used in the 'gold standard', safest HRT, along with estrogen.

Progestins, on the other hand, are synthesised from testosterone, and sometimes from progesterone itself, but they have a different chemical structure from natural progesterone. Progestins are used in almost all contraceptive pills, and most of the older forms of combined HRT, which tended to cause small increases in breast cancer.[30] I hated being on the combined contraceptive pill: it flattened me and my sex drive, and the low mood and weight gain that some women experience on the pill is often a reaction to synthetic progestins. 'Progestin and progesterone have the same beneficial thinning effect on the uterine lining but almost opposite effects in every other part of the body including the breasts and brain,' says Dr Lara Briden, author of the *Hormone Repair Manual*. 'That's why progesterone is safer than a progestin and also has fewer side effects for mood and even hair.'[31] The fact that this difference is so often ignored has been called out as sloppy science[32] that has given *all* HRT a bad rap.

What we can say with some certainty about progesterone is that during the perimenopause it goes haywire. While proceeding in a general downward direction from the age of 40 in most women and flatlining at around 50, it can have peaks and troughs on the way, but the major effect of its decline on women is an increase in anxiety and insomnia. I tried to find out if there was a peak in numbers of people googling the word 'perimenopause' at 3 a.m. and 4 a.m., but there were no statistics. What I did find, on Google Trends, was that searches for 'perimenopause' have quadrupled in the past ten years. The interest in progesterone has grown, too, but not in progestins. I suspect, like me, that the 70 per cent of women that have ever used the contraceptive pill had no idea exactly what they were putting in the bodies, and most still have no idea what is in HRT. Arming ourselves with that knowledge is essential to our future health.

Testosterone

Last but not least is testosterone, a hormone that women must start to reclaim for themselves. The story of testosterone begins with a famously ballsy moment in 1889, when the 72-year-old French scientist Charles Édouard Brown-Séquard injected himself with liquid from the testicles of a dog (or possibly a guinea pig – records are unclear) daily for three weeks. He found not just improved energy, muscle strength and a magnificent 'jet of urine', but also a subjective enhancement of his brain power, as he wrote scientific papers into the night.[33] A few weeks after ending his injections, he returned to 'a state of weakness'. Brown-Séquard may have been completely barking, but his research was the start of the twentieth-century race to understand male testosterone: the Greek God hormone, the 'Elixir of Life', the alchemy that makes a man a man.

But it turns out that testosterone also makes a woman a woman – and a sexy and smart woman at that. As I've mentioned before, testosterone is the hormone women produce in the largest quantity, followed by estrogen and progesterone.[34] While men lose testosterone on a slope as they age, female hormones tend to fall off the cliff at the menopause. When our ovaries slow production of all three hormones around the menopause, for some lucky women a bit of testosterone remains, and it continues to gently decline through their sixties and even seventies. It's often the last hormone standing, and thus gains dominance.

But many find the testosterone bank is empty. Mine was, according to a blood test. We normally have about a tenth of the testosterone of a man, yet knowledge of its powerful effect on women is over a century behind. The latest hormone research emerging shows that while estrogen is the petrol in the female car, testosterone may well be the spark plugs. 'Just because there's more testosterone in men than women, more doesn't mean more important, and size isn't always everything,' said Lauren Redfern, an anthropologist at the London School of Hygiene & Tropical Medicine, whose *Rethinking Testosterone* PhD project is exploring the use of testosterone in the UK from both patients' and professionals' perspectives.

Testosterone is a trump hormone for women, and I mean that in a good way. We have testosterone receptors in all the important sites, including our brains, breasts and vulvas. Testosterone is not just about libido; studies of mice and men show it increases energy, cognitive power, memory, muscle and bone strength.[35] Some women with low natural levels of testosterone experience depressive moods, brain fog and fatigue, as well as decreased sex drive. Dr Shahzadi Harper was an NHS GP for over 20 years before deciding to become a private menopause specialist in London, and now considers testosterone as part of each consultation. 'Women take estrogen and progesterone first, but some still find that their oomph is missing and testosterone is the missing piece of the jigsaw,' she explained. 'Your fat-to-muscle ratio changes when you have testosterone. For sex, brain, energy and body shape testosterone really matters, and there's even a case for some women starting it in perimenopause. It just brings women back to normal.'

Testosterone has a mighty role in the female sex drive as well as the male. According to a British Menopause Society survey, 51 per cent of women say the menopause adversely affects their sex life,[36] and it's the fall in testosterone that's to blame for these languishing libidos. Your testosterone at 40 years old is about half of that at 20, and continues to decline during the menopause. This is not helped by the disappearance of estrogen around the vulva, which can make sex painful. (There's a whole chapter to come on rescuing your vagina and sex life, and maintaining both far into the future.) At the same time, women in midlife are often offered antidepressants, and SSRI antidepressants, in particular, are notorious for being 'orgasm blockers', causing sexual dysfunction in both men and women. Many women also seem to accept the loss of solo or accompanied sex as a part of growing older, and some embrace celibacy as a new freedom.

Others, like the writer Rowan Pelling, founder of the literary and erotic magazine *The Erotic Review*, believe 'there is no pleasure greater than sexual intimacy'; Pelling continues: 'I will cling to the flame while there's the tiniest red ember in the grate.' I had a long discussion with the 54-year-old, whose Twitter description is 'Born a barmaid, plans to perish in an over-laced corset.' She was enraged by the sexism surrounding testosterone, and plans to get a prescription for herself if her famed appetite begins to falter. 'This is what I'm hearing from my friends – it has a miraculous effect on desire.' She believes women who want to beat a retreat from the erotic arena should be supported, too. 'I totally understand why some friends feel delighted to be unshackled from the demands of an unruly sex drive, and find that gardening, cooking and dancing give them more joy. But it's a national scandal that we don't prioritise older women's rights to a decent sex life, but almost any bloke who asks can get his mitts on Viagra.'

The NHS provides men with around 3 million prescriptions of Viagra (or the non-branded sildenafil) every year in the UK,[37] as one in five experience erectile dysfunction. Around 20 per cent of men also have lower-than-normal testosterone, and can have that tested and topped up on the NHS. *Straightaway, Sir! Something for the weekend, Sir?* So, while men in their fifties are chemically and hormonally primed for action by our health service, neglected women with low libidos and painful vaginas are downing tools, except those of the gardening sort. This disparity often results in diminished intimacy in relationships or even midlife divorce.

Why are the medical rules and cultural assumptions so different for men and women around the sex hormone that they both have? Why were we wrongly taught in secondary schools, and even many medical schools (according to many doctors I've interviewed), that estrogen is the female hormone and testosterone is the male, and never the twain shall meet? It also turns out that men need estrogen too, to complete their hormonal cocktail.

For now, however, the mainstream scientific struggle around testosterone remains binary and simplistic. As Lauren Redfern argues, 'the idea that science and technology is truth, is in itself biased. We start research because we have hypotheses. Testosterone studies have all been about the gendered idea of being a man, the fighting and fucking hormone, and hegemonic male aggression. There's very limited research on women, and I was drawn to that.' Redfern explains that testosterone's effects on the female body are different from those on the male. 'The only way I can put it into context is petrol in a car – the same substance works differently in every machine, with different responses.' In Cordelia Fine's book *Testosterone Rex*, the author also laments the simplistic, men-only portrayal of testosterone. 'It misrepresents our past, present and future; it misdirects scientific research; and it reinforces an unequal status quo. It's time to say goodbye, and move on.'[38] Assumptions about hormones are also becoming more fluid as the voice of the trans and non-binary movement grows.

Whether or not testosterone is inherent or supplemented, we need to know more about it, whether to understand ourselves in seed-sowing youth, in the wild throes of the perimenopause or in the empowered aftermath of the menopause. Testosterone is not yet part of women's everyday vocabulary, but it has always played a big part in female lives, being the principal hormone that continues to be produced by the adrenal glands after the menopause (if you're lucky). The women who say they 'sail through' the menopause are probably the ones floating on a sea of their own testosterone, maintaining energy, sex drive, memory and strength. Many have a surge of energy and brilliant careers after the menopause – I keep thinking of the US Supreme Court lawyer Ruth Bader Ginsberg, who worked tirelessly for legal equality until she died at 87, still on the bench; or all the grannies hauling buggies and toddlers for mothers and fathers who are out working; or my friend Margaret, who is in her nineties and continuing her academic education on Zoom, and who told me, 'Oh, the menopause gave me no trouble at all, dear. In fact, I had a real burst of energy afterwards. Later, a new path gradually opened out and I am most grateful for it.'

When that culturally embedded female desire to please just drops away, battle begins and freedom beckons. Even though I've still got some estrogen coursing through my blood, I feel that I no longer need to be pliable or polite just to fit in. Perhaps that's the testosterone, or perhaps that's the wisdom of midlife, but honesty is now my only policy. Author Darcey Steinke explains that her menopause enabled her to slip out from under a 'claustrophobic femininity'.[39] She is not, she writes, 'fully masculine', either, but feels 'in the middle, a third gender'. She adds: 'I'm 57 now; my symptoms are less. I also think I've gotten used to it. Instead of feeling disoriented outside of the cycle, I feel that it's a very freeing, beautiful time.'

Steinke's book is a beautifully written paean to the pain and glory of natural menopause, unaided by hormones, and I believe women should support rather than judge each other as we make our individual journeys into midlife. In Steinke's studies on orcas, mentioned in Chapter 1, it turns out – from 'blubber biopsies' on living premenopausal whales – that females have exceptionally high concentrations of testosterone.[40] We don't yet know what happens to their hormones after the menopause, but I await any future research on 'granny' whales with interest.

When the nurturing mother-hormones estrogen and progesterone die away and testosterone becomes dominant, the small amount of remaining testosterone can predispose some women to androgenic symptoms such as acne, increased facial hair growth and male-pattern baldness. These are usually minor, and the upside is power, drive and ambition. (Incidentally, I haven't grown a single stray chin-hair, and I use testosterone every morning in the amounts that were in my body pre-menopause.) The pioneering twentieth-century cape-wearing anthropologist Margaret Mead described a 'physical and psychological surge of energy' in her fifties and worked until her late seventies, concluding that: 'There is no more creative force in the world than a menopausal woman with zest.' (She also persuaded her doctor to give her estrogen injections back in 1949, but seemingly had no need to top up her own testosterone.) Mead gave us the term 'postmenopausal zest', PMZ, a superpower after all those miserable years of PMS.

For women, particularly those of us who will work full-time until retirement age at 67 or longer, and will live on average into our eighties, testosterone is not a lifestyle drug but a life-saving hormone that will preserve our brains, bodies and long-term health. Lauren Redfern differentiates treatment for enhancement for sports or muscle-building and treatment for prevention: 'I myself think the postmenopausal use of testosterone is about prevention and protection.' Most women are not super-powered athletes overdosing on testosterone to run extreme triathlons. Instead, they are replacing depleted hormones so they can work long hours as nurses, business executives and key workers on the till at Tesco, and they also want to keep their relationships alive. Testosterone should not be an afterthought, but one of the first solutions for struggling menopausal women. The well-being expert and Menopause Charity ambassador Liz Earle also uses testosterone and describes it as 'part of the Holy Trinity of female hormones'.

The experts agree. 'There is irrefutable evidence of testosterone's effect on increased sexual function in women,[41] but we need a bigger study on the role of testosterone in women in the prevention of diseases of ageing, including cardiovascular disease, and its effect on bone density and cognition,' says Professor Susan Davis, former president of the International Menopause Society and an endocrinologist at Monash University in Melbourne, Australia. Thanks partly to Davis's groundbreaking research and advocacy, AndroFeme testosterone cream for women – which comes in a reassuring pink, toothpaste-like tube – was licensed in 2020 throughout the Australian health system, and the British Menopause Society and The Menopause Charity are campaigning for the cream to be licensed here on the NHS. First Vegemite, next AndroFeme.

What's even more fascinating is Davis's research into the effect of testosterone on the menopausal female brain. Many studies have already shown that testosterone supplementation improves memory and spatial cognition in older men,[42] but women have been left out of the research picture. In a randomised controlled trial, Davis and her colleagues tested testosterone gel and a placebo gel on 92 menopausal women who were not already on HRT. The hormone gel elevated serum testosterone levels into the normal range for premenopausal women. The trial reported: 'Our consistent and specific finding of improved performance on tests of verbal learning and memory with testosterone therapy . . . suggests a contribution of testosterone to verbal memory in post-menopausal women.'[43] In laywoman's terms, after 26 weeks on testosterone, the women remembered many more items on a simple shopping list – and no one grew hairy. Davis is encouraged by the results but thinks we need bigger trials. Research money is not yet forthcoming.

My own one-woman experiment in returning my testosterone to normal, premenopausal levels correlates with Davis's research on verbal memory. Aside from hot flushes and hair loss, it was my short-circuiting memory that finally pushed me to search for safe HRT. I realised what was happening on an ordinary Saturday morning when I thought, 'I must shave my legs,' and went to write a shopping list. I wrote down 'shaver' because I couldn't remember the word 'razor'. I stood there in the kitchen, staring the list, knowing it was wrong, panicking. I'd occasionally forgotten people's names before – I had a job that entailed watching 350 films a year, so losing a supporting-actor credit wasn't surprising, given the encyclopaedic load. But this was a completely different sort of memory loss. Razor was an everyday noun. And because my mother had died of Alzheimer's disease, shedding nouns from her vocabulary over the years like confetti, I was terrified – and alone, scared to tell anyone what was happening.

The solution, fortunately, was simple. Soon after taking testosterone coupled with estrogen – which has an equally powerful effect on the brain – my memory returned. I felt the dark shroud of Alzheimer's slither off my shoulders, and the first thing I wanted to do was get the good news out to other anxious women who thought they were losing their memories and minds – the whole of Chapter 11 is dedicated to the menopausal brain and Alzheimer's.

Just being aware of your hormones' protective superpowers, and their erratically descending levels in the perimenopause and menopause, is reassuring. But once you know the reason symptoms and changes are occurring, the question of how to deal with them arises, and solutions are at hand in the upcoming chapters on HRT and alternative remedies (Chapters 8 and 7 respectively). You may be behaving strangely in midlife, but you are no longer alone . . .

After my own testosterone boost, I asked three women already on basic HRT to add testosterone for the second Davina McCall documentary. 'The brain fog was worst. I forgot names and I'd be looking at someone and the name had gone,' said Paula Fry, a City executive. I wanted solid evidence, so I asked the women to rate 20 menopause symptoms, including brain fog, energy and libido, and complete memory tests. After two months, the changes were encouraging: 'I seem to have a sharpness back, a real clarity about what I'm trying to say,' said Joanne Harding, a councillor. Maggie Dennis, a manager, said: 'I can remember my husband's mobile number!' And Fry said, 'it just feels like a lift in mood, the missing piece of the jigsaw'.

4

THE MENOPAUSE AT WORK

Of all the hard-working people in the world, the ones we needed most in the tough, wintry months of the Covid-19 pandemic were nurses, most of whom, in the UK, are women, and half of whom are of menopausal age. My friend Jasmine, whom I've known since our children were at nursery school together, is a nursing sister in the obstetrics and gynaecology department at one of the busiest London hospitals. As the pandemic gathered pace, she ended up working three twelve-hour shifts a week in ob-gyn and three more twelve-hour shifts on the Covid-19 vaccination team, inoculating 45–50 patients a day. She found the work incredibly satisfying, and said to me at the time: 'They're so happy – they thank you like you invented the vaccine yourself.' But the 72-hour week took its toll, not to mention the febrile, panicked atmosphere in the hospital and the unceasing sirens. 'They're asking anyone who can to go and work in the intensive care unit,' she said. 'Maybe I should go?' But she sounded completely shattered. Any normal human might find her work schedule burdensome, but at 49,

Jasmine was in the middle of the perimenopause, or possibly the menopause – she didn't know which. 'I can't tell where I am any more because I haven't had periods for years since I use a Mirena [hormonal] coil. I just know it's chaos.'

I thought she was doing more than enough, vaccinating 150 people a week and holding down her other job; she didn't need to spend her one day off in the ICU. Jasmine needed to look after herself properly, and consequently the NHS. 'I keep bursting into tears,' she said. 'I thought I was going to cry as I was vaccinating a patient. But I went away and washed my face. I held on until I got home.'

This was not like Jasmine: she is down-to-earth, funny, kind and could run a small country if necessary. She had always coped with the stress of working in the NHS; indeed, she loves her job. But, like me, in her late forties she had sudden, unexpected heart palpitations so her GP sent her for an electrocardiogram – and didn't even discuss the impending menopause. The cardiogram results were absolutely fine. 'Classic perimenopause symptom,' I told her, recounting the medical studies showing how common it was.[1] But Jasmine wasn't getting any hot flushes (though she'd had a few previously) and thought things had settled down. She was reluctant to consider HRT, and perhaps reluctant, like I was, to face the fact she was going through either the perimenopause or the menopause. When she went back to the GP again, her doctor was happy to prescribe antidepressants, but less keen on hormone replacement.

Jasmine's symptoms piled up – hair loss, a low-level depression and sleepless nights riddled with unnamed anxiety. She told me she'd been in a job interview and forgotten an essential phrase. It was, appropriately, 'occupational health'. 'I don't know what's happened to my memory,' she said to me one day. Jasmine had been a stalwart confidante throughout my own menopausal crash as well as my divorce, so she'd heard it all before, yet like all of us, she found it hard to look after her own health. 'And you're a nurse!' I admonished her. Then one day, when Covid hospital admissions were at their peak, Jasmine rang and said she had gone in desperation to a private gynaecologist she knew and had her hormone levels measured: they were incredibly low. 'I've got it!' she rejoiced. 'I've got some estrogen gel!'

Because Jasmine hadn't been sure if she was menopausal, despite her symptoms, she hadn't felt confident about discussing HRT with her GP again. She had been sent away twice before without hormonal help, and she hadn't considered asking the GP to put her on the waiting list for the local NHS menopause clinic – which, ironically, turned out to be *in the same hospital* where she worked. But once she'd been prescribed HRT by the private doctor, the improvement was instantaneous: 'I just slept the whole night through. I couldn't believe it.' Jasmine's anxiety diminished too, despite being on the pandemic frontline. 'I don't feel up and down any more. I'm much more optimistic,' she said a few weeks later. 'I feel I'm looking in a whole new direction, into the next part of my life.' For a while she even became the family liaison officer on the Covid ICU, a job that required wisdom and emotional resilience.

Information about the perimenopause and menopause just wasn't easily available to Jasmine, even in a workplace run by the NHS. Her GP wasn't fully informed and the subject had barely been given a mention in her own medical training. A symptom-list poster on the hospital bathroom wall might have helped; a training session for managers; a workshop for employees; a simple health check; a lecture for all staff from the experts at the in-house menopause clinic. In fact, shouldn't preparing women for the menopause be part of . . . occupational health?

Right now, the menopause causes an omnishambles in the workplace, as capable women like Jasmine are left without medical support or advice from Human Resources and are flummoxed by their own symptoms – in Jasmine's case, she didn't know most of them were menopausal until *after* she took HRT. With that in mind, I helped create a Channel 4/Fawcett Society survey[2] on menopause in the workplace for the Davina McCall documentary – the biggest ever done in the UK. We questioned 4,000 diverse perimenopausal and menopausal women aged 45-55, and discovered that an astounding one in ten had left their jobs due to symptoms. *One in ten.* What a waste of mature, experienced workers. What a cost to lives – and the economy. And there was more: around 14 per cent had gone part time, and another 14 per cent said they had cut their hours – more so for disabled women. Almost half surveyed said symptoms had affected their ability to do their job, and eight per cent had not applied for promotion. Women were self-censoring, and 52 per cent said they had lost confidence. And it's not just in the UK. An international survey of 700 working women in Australia, the USA and UK by Circle In[3] which supports employees revealed that almost half said they had experienced a 'drop in confidence' due to the menopause, and 46 per cent cited the constant stress of hiding their symptoms from management.

The 'don't ask, don't tell' attitude to the menopause does neither employers nor employees any favours. The fact is that nine out of ten menopausal women say symptoms have had a negative effect on their work[4] and that they wouldn't tell their employer the real reason why they were taking a sick day;[5] the most common reason cited on a sickness certificate by women with menopausal symptoms is 'anxiety or stress'. We can't even statistically track the problem – because on paper it doesn't exist.

Women between 45 and 55 make up 11 per cent of the workforce in industrialised countries and global menopause productivity loss has been estimated at £110 billion a year.[6] How devastating is this loss of staff, experience and time for organisations? Let's just look more closely at the NHS, where 50 per cent of nurses are over 50 years old and where, as a Royal College of Nursing survey showed, one third of nurses were considering leaving, due to low pay and their treatment during the pandemic.[7] 'We're facing a time bomb,' says Karen Storey, who is the National Primary Care Nursing Lead for NHS England and works with NHS Improvement to advance patient care and leadership. 'There's burnout, there's exhaustion and there's menopause, too. A third of our workforce could leave or retire. Some nurses can take early retirement with their pensions at 55.' All that expensive training – and empathy – could be tossed away like a used cardboard bedpan, unless experienced nurses are given the respect and support they deserve. As my friend Jasmine pointed out, she could take a two-day private course called 'Botox and Dermal Fillers Training for Nurses and Midwives' and change to a less stressful, better-paid job. But Jasmine has a vocation, not just a job, and now that she's feeling healthy, she's sticking with it.

I had hoped that at least doctors themselves would be informed and vocal about menopause in the workplace, but it turns out the adage 'Physician, heal thyself' does not apply to the menopause. Female doctors have nightmarish struggles with their own menopauses, or at least the 2,000 who answered a British Medical Association survey do.[8] What was astonishing was how helpless they all seemed to feel when faced with the transition. Eighty-three per cent said symptoms had impacted their working lives, a third wanted to change their jobs, and there was a pattern of experienced doctors taking a step back in their careers, moving to easier, lower-paid roles and leaving positions as clinical leaders or directors. Only 16 per cent had discussed their symptoms with a manager. As one doctor explained: 'There are very few older women left at my senior level in my traditional profession. If I mentioned my perimenopausal symptoms, I would be stigmatised and disrespected as someone who was no longer rational or capable.'

What world are we living in that doctors are afraid to talk about their own mental and physical health? The high-pressure, macho work ethic in medicine seems to be life-and soul-destroying for the women in the BMA survey, who were aged between 45 and 55, and there are 30,000 doctors in that age group in the UK. Sadly, the women felt the unsupportive culture came not just from management, but even from peers. Many talked about the impact on their mental health. Overwhelmed by sleeplessness and from being on call, a few started to doubt their abilities. One doctor confessed: 'I am quite happy to talk about my physical symptoms, as my boss is a woman who has been through the menopause. My hormone-related mental-health issues are more complex and, when I'm experiencing them, I don't feel able to talk to anyone, let alone ask for changes I feel I don't deserve, as I appear to be doing my job so badly. I suffer attacks of low confidence, which makes me question my worth and ability to do my job. When coupled with the symptoms, I have often felt like giving up.'

The killer symptoms most affecting work are hot flushes, experienced by 80 per cent of women,[9] along with memory lapses and disturbed sleep, leading to fatigue and poor concentration. Aside from the secret discomfort and sometimes public humiliation of suddenly sweating, hot flushes cause temporary lows in glucose, which feeds the brain. 'Hot flushes have previously been considered a bothersome but benign symptom of menopause,'[10] said Professor Pauline Maki of the Center for Research on Women and Gender at the University of Illinois at Chicago. But her 2020 study testing the recall abilities of 14 menopausal women shows that hot flushes are not 'power surges', as they are often referred to, but power outages. 'There was a direct association between objectively measured hot flushes, memory difficulties and alterations in memory circuits in women's brains.'[11] Basically, as blood rushes to the surface of your body during a hot flush, the blood flow to your brain goes down, by 5 per cent or more. Each flush lasts an average of four minutes, and your focus is often more on the discomfort that the task in hand.[12] Unsurprisingly, your PowerPoint presentation can go down the plughole. More numerous hot flushes resulted in worse verbal memory on immediate tests and recall later on. New research discussed in Chapter 11 shows that memory does recover in around 80 per cent of women, as brains rewire in the years post-menopause and hot flushes eventually come to an end – although some women suffer flushes into their eighties. In the meantime, though, finding ways to calm those hot spikes is important, and HRT, cannabidiol capsules, eating soy products, giving up alcohol, cognitive behavioural therapy and even certain antidepressants may help with overheating.

The temporary wipeout of a hot flush is worsened for many by ongoing brain fog caused by estrogen receptors in the brain already being starved of fuel. A friend of mine from university, now an experienced and empathetic secondary school teacher, sent me a poignant WhatsApp message about her own brain fog after I told her about this book when we reconnected during the long evenings of the Covid-19 epidemic. 'This lockdown is also making me feel stupid . . . because it's underlining my inability to learn new computer teaching tricks. I've already been passed over in the department for someone younger because she can use a computer better than me. Of course she bloody can! Some days I sit for a frantic 20 minutes trying to remember my password – I write it down, I forget where, I cry – am I starting to lose it? Other days I'm in . . . then I can't transfer an image to duplicate it and save it somewhere else . . . All I've done, my years of experience, are for nothing – this damn wee square screen is going to be the end of me. I think many women are going to come out of this crisis into a worse personal crisis . . . if they come out at all. So what do we do? We reach for the wine.'

There is a multipronged assault going on here. Rapidly changing technology, but no rapid training in it; younger colleagues coming up; women losing career traction due to pregnancy and parenting; and menopausal women being seen as 'past their peak' while men in their fifties are generally seen as reliably mature. Plus, there's the upsetting experience of genuine, if temporary, memory loss, which kicks a hole in your confidence. Actually, my friend made a comeback after those gruelling early days, once she got on top of the technology and could communicate and connect with her pupils, and her experience shone through. We are magnificent creatures in midlife, and we should not forget that we have human-handling skills forged in fire over the years, and that we at last have time to dedicate to jobs or projects beyond our grown families. Simply not shopping and cooking and washing for, say, four other people every day can suddenly give you an hour to think and create. Those most basic domestic duties take up at least seven hours a week – almost a whole working day regained for your life or your career. Yet so many brilliant women I know have more time now but are struggling at work, where employer acknowledgement of many of these challenging symptoms, coupled with medical advice, would make most of these troubles melt away.

Some careers can be destroyed by menopause symptoms that are left untreated. I heard about a soprano at one a major opera company whose vocal range completely changed with the menopause. Her voice became dry and less flexible, and she was unable to properly reach the highest notes. Voice retraining can sometimes help here, but she was sent for a vocal review and was on the verge of losing her job. She decided to try HRT, and after three months on estrogen her voice came back, her vocal cords responded correctly and she hit her high notes. She also felt much better. There are some fascinating medical papers out there on this, including one sonorously titled 'The Voice and Menopause: The Twilight of the Divas'.[13]

The majority of women have to keep working alongside these irritating symptoms every day. Most cope magnificently through the years of hormonal fluctuations and continue with their lives and careers, but discussion and some small-scale adjustments – to uniforms, to flexible working, to room temperature, to bathroom breaks – might make a big difference in the retention of experienced, qualified female staff. The sudden, flooding periods of the perimenopause and increased urinary tract niggles of the menopause are also hard to handle when shifts are inflexible and access to restrooms inconvenient. If you are, say, one of the growing number of workers packing orders for home delivery from big warehouses, long bathroom breaks may be considered 'time off task'[14] and can result in questioning from your manager. The campaign to change the law to allow flexible working for everyone from day one, launched in 2021 by the Chartered Institute of Personnel and Development,[15] might help women cope with those difficult days and make up the time elsewhere. The Advisory, Conciliation and Arbitration Service (ACAS), too, suggests that if a worker is off sick due to the perimenopause or menopause, the employer should record these absences differently so they are not unfairly measured as part of the worker's overall attendance record.

'It's important that employers and managers understand that the menopause is a natural life event, not an illness,' says Sarah Davies, a former business manager who set up the menopause-at-work training programme Talking Menopause[16] to educate staff in companies and public organisations about the menopause. 'The stigma and taboo around menopause stops women discussing it at work.' But if employers thought of menopause the same way they think of pregnancy – not a disability, or an illness, but a period in a woman's life where some flexibility, empathy and practical help would make it possible to continue working – the problem might be swiftly solved. Davies has run workshop sessions for supermarkets such as ASDA, for police forces such as those in Avon and Dorset, and the security and defence contractor Qinetiq. 'We find a quarter of working women have severe symptoms – and three-quarters of those don't even realise their symptoms are due to the menopause.'

But the law around the menopause is changing. 'Employers also need to understand that menopause discrimination can now be a legal issue,' explains Deborah Garlick, founder of the menopause-at-work advisory company Henpicked. 'Menopause symptoms can give rise to a Section 6 Equality Act 2010 disability, provided the symptoms have a long-term adverse effect on normal activities.' The first case won on menopause-related disability was *Ms M. Davies v. Scottish Courts and Tribunals*, in 2018.[17] Davies was being treated for the perimenopause, urinary tract infections and flooding periods by her doctor, and during that time she was sacked as a court officer after making a mistake due to menopausal forgetfulness. The tribunal said this was unfair dismissal due to disability and she was reinstated and awarded £20,000 compensation. I'm not sure that the menopause should be classed as a legal disability, but the Equality Act 2010 also deals with pregnancy and maternity discrimination, so perhaps menopause discrimination could eventually be added to that list. In the 2012 case *Merchant v. British Telecommunications*, a tribunal said direct sex discrimination had occurred when an employer had failed to treat an employee's menopause like other medical conditions. When it was suggested that

Merchant, the defendant, was underperforming, she provided her employers with a letter from her GP that said that the menopause 'can affect her level of concentration at times'. Employers beware. 'Consider the potential reputation costs, too,' says Garlick.

One of the best ways to avoid conflict and staff losses is to create a menopause policy. This isn't rocket science, and there are plenty of examples. Henpicked has a good selection for employers,[18] and most begin with providing menopause awareness, information on symptoms, and support for employees and managers of all genders. They policies then look at difficult work conditions and the possibility of making 'reasonable adjustments' to uniforms or hours, so women feel comfortable. The campaigning Welsh Labour MP Carolyn Harris has promoted mandatory menopause policies in Parliament, and in October 2021 won cross-party support to make HRT prescriptions subject to a one-off annual charge in England (they are already free in Scotland and Wales). Harris said: 'Women should not feel inferior or incapable of doing their job because of the effects of the menopause on their health and well-being, but, sadly, too many do. The situation could be so easily rectified.'

Having a written menopause policy and some public cheerleading can really make a difference, and companies like Sainsbury's, Next, Tesco, Marks & Spencer, John Lewis, Aviva, Southeastern railways, as well as many universities and NHS trusts, are leading the way. But smaller workplaces and the private, non-unionised sector may lag behind. The Channel 4/Fawcett Survey discovered the eight out of ten workplaces had no menopause policy or training, and

23 per cent of key workers say their uniform makes them uncomfortable.[19] A Trades Union Congress survey revealed only 1 per cent of women knew their workplace had a menopause policy – 46 per cent said that no policy existed in their workplace and the remaining 53 per cent had no idea.[20] Talking Menopause's Sarah Davies explains: 'When we go into companies, we find that women are afraid to speak up about their own symptoms and ask for help. Productivity levels fall dramatically and absenteeism increases, both having a direct impact on profit levels – never mind on the women themselves.'

Putting decency, inclusivity and kindness aside – which often happens in the job market – the argument for giving menopausal employees the care they deserve is a rock-solid economic one. *The Economist* and the *Financial Times* have started covering the subject with interest. The loss of talent and experience when women move on is immeasurable, but the loss of time can be quantified. One survey of 1,000 women aged between 50 and 64 revealed that a third had taken an average of three days off per year due to symptoms.[21] That's a potential productivity loss, across the UK female workforce, of 14 million working days.

In fact, menopausal women are the fastest-growing group of workers in the UK economy, as retirement age rises and more women work later in life – there are now 4.5 million of us.[22] During the Covid-19 pandemic, female key workers were the titans holding the frontline: women make up 77 per cent of NHS employees, 63 per cent of supermarket workers and 47 per cent of the total workforce.[23] Almost all will experience the perimenopause and menopause for about 20 years while on the job. The average woman will work 16 years after the menopause, retiring at 67, and those of us with rubbish pensions (or none at all) will work longer. Yet this golden age, after tough years of intense parenting, should be a time for midlife women, as it is for men, to consolidate their careers and have their wisdom and experience valued and promoted. On the whole, though, it's not. Temporary, menopausal blips can have long-term consequences, when simple discussion and acceptance of the menopause in the workspace could stop that. Many women do not need time off, but making small allowances for symptoms would help – as would making sure that women have time to visit a doctor and are properly informed of their choices.

We are still battling a bulwark of negativity about the menopause in working culture. When the deputy governor of the Bank of England, Ben Broadbent, described the faltering UK economy as 'menopausal' in a newspaper interview, saying it was 'past its peak and no longer potent',[24] that opened a very public window into the disdain for older women everywhere, and particularly in the workplace. Broadbent's remark was rounded on for its sexism, and when he apologised, explaining he was comparing the economy now to the 'climacteric' period at the end of the nineteenth century, when the Age of Steam was running out of steam, that just made things worse.

After this new low in mansplaining, academic and television presenter Mary Beard said: 'The idea that the adjective "menopausal" can be used as a description for "economic slump" is something of an ideological give-away (and guaranteed to prompt a strong reaction from those millions of us 50-plus-year-old women who don't feel we are slumping). How long have we had to argue that being past childbearing is not like being past one's sell-by date, as if fertility was women's only purpose? I could go on![25]

We need to tackle the menopause from a medical *and* cultural standpoint in the workplace, where banter can make things worse. Sexist jokes abound: 'Q: Why do women stop bleeding after the menopause? A: Because they need the blood for their varicose veins.' Or 'Q: How do you know your fridge is going through the menopause? A: It's all out of eggs.' In the TUC survey of menopausal women, six out of ten had witnessed the issue being treated as a joke in the workplace.[26] But women themselves bear some of the blame for the comedy culture when they enter into what I call 'menopause masochism' and perpetuate the clichés. Perhaps black humour around the menopause helps older women bond, or cope with unnecessary shame around the menopause, but personally I want to smash the novelty tea-break mugs that say *I'm still hot – but it just comes in flashes* and rip down the office posters saying, *What are the names of the seven menopausal dwarves? Itchy, Bitchy, Sweaty, Sleepy, Bloated, Forgetful and Psycho.* We're not doing ourselves any favours by joking about the menopause – or hiding it.

A big, noisy conversation about the menopause gives women confidence, and makes it easier for male colleagues, too. West Midlands Police have made huge strides in normalising the menopause amongst frontline and support staff. After all, who wants to get a hot flush while wearing a heavy stab-proof vest and jacket while driving to an emergency? My knowledge of middle-aged female policing was entirely based on Sarah Lancashire's fictional character in TV's *Happy Valley,* so I wanted to know more. I met Chief Inspector Yvonne Bruton in a concrete behemoth of a building in Birmingham, appropriate to the might of the force – around 10,000 police officers, just over a third of whom are women, plus support staff. Chief Inspector Bruton runs the Women in Policing group. 'The impact of the menopause on the organisation is huge if women are up three times a night, never mind the impact on partners and family. If female officers were finding it hard out on a 999 call as single crew, then we can make sure they have a buddy. And if an officer has to stand on scene for hours, we can make sure they get a toilet break. We ask about mental health and well-being. We have a 'reasonable adjustment passport' which outlines each woman's needs, from chairs to working hours, and that passport stays with them when they move departments and is reviewed regularly.'

Bruton's civilian colleague Carol Brown runs a regular menopause support group for policewomen, and the pair arranged a workshop for female officers run by the training organisation Laughology. 'We had a stand-up comedian come in to break the ice and talk about the menopause in the evening with women and their husbands or partners.' While derogatory humour is damaging, humour used sensitively and compassionately around the menopause can aid understanding. West Midlands Police is also keen to debunk the myths about HRT, and brings in doctors to talk to staff, as well as supplying leaflets and posters. Bruton says the policy change has improved retention of middle-aged policewomen, with valuable results: 'Keeping that experience equals an excellent policing service.' Chief Inspector Bruton also heads the West Midlands force's Violence Reduction Unit, and notes that domestic violence can often peak around the menopause.

Women who are already battered by mood swings and other symptoms can find that conflict escalates, and men can suffer domestic violence, too. An understanding, experienced officer can make a big difference when they knock on the door.

The improvements at West Midlands Police could be mirrored countrywide if changes being discussed by Carolyn Harris's parliamentary group succeed – mandatory workplace menopause policies and increased information and access to menopause healthcare. In Australia, the Future Super ethical investment company, half of whose staff are female, has introduced a menstrual and menopause leave policy that allows workers to take up to six days off a year, which are not counted as sick leave. The UK still awaits such acknowledgement.

I've been writing here about menopause misery – and rescue – at work, but there is, of course, a wonderful alternative universe out there where menopausal women make fulfilling decisions to change career, return to education, volunteer or live a less stressful life after children have left home, and my own midlife reboot has been exhilarating as well as tricky. For the privileged, with money in the bank, making a leap to another career is a risk worth taking, an empowering re-envisioning. But for most women it's not quite so easy, yet knowing there's a growing community out there on social media, and on podcasts like *Postcards from Midlife*, brings courage.

Eleanor Mills was an editor at the *Sunday Times* for 23 years, until she took redundancy and founded the midlife 'pivot' site Noon, which empowers women to take charge and make change. 'The collision of ageism and sexism sees women in midlife sidelined at work,' she says. 'It is the point where women become more confident but also less malleable and "pleasing" to men on many levels. How unsurprising that many women are deemed surplus to requirements.' Aside from bias towards youthful beauty, is midlife women's new-found confidence another reason why television presenters and actresses find work drying up and female executives hit the hormonal ceiling? Do some powerful male executives still secretly prefer their female colleagues, however smart, to be flirty and fertile rather than challenging and confident? Mills says: 'There's a certain kind of boss that likes his female deputies to do a bit of ego fluffing – never mind the other sort of fluffing – and when you're too old or wise to provide that service, when you have the confidence to confront when it matters, you get dropped.'

Menopause concealment is a crime many of us have committed, just to stay in the game. For women in their late forties and fifties, mentioning the menopause is like admitting to a sell-by date, and is instantly ageing in the eyes of old-fashioned bosses. I never, ever mentioned the menopause at work, or let any of my symptoms affect me professionally; I never missed a deadline. The crazy perimenopausal stuff happened at home instead. But in 2017, after 26 stimulating years at *The Times* – on contract as an interviewer and foreign columnist in Paris, New York and Washington, and latterly on staff as chief film critic – I felt I had to move on. In my job, I was increasingly incensed by the lack of diversity and representation for women on screen, back when 95 per cent of mainstream movies were directed by white men. (That's starting to change for the better now.) I had a growing feminist Twitter following, @muirkate, campaigned with Women and Hollywood, which agitates for gender diversity and inclusion in the global film industry, and stirred up trouble when women were sent away for refusing to wear high heels on the red carpet at Cannes.[27] Increasingly, I wanted to feel free to say and do anything I liked, beyond traditional journalism.

To my surprise, leaving *The Times* turned out to be one of the best things that's ever happened to me. I don't know if it was a postmenopausal reawakening, but I studied at the London Film School part-time and learned to write television scripts, which became the catalyst for the Davina McCall menopause documentaries. I started a novel set in Victorian Glasgow. I rebuilt a damp, subsiding terraced house that had been lived in for 50 years by Peter Baldwin, who played Derek in *Coronation Street* before he died; old scripts from the soap rained out of long-locked cupboards. I felt like I'd come home, in every sense. And when the Time's Up UK movement had its first meeting, in London in early 2018, I joined it to work on the representation of critics and screenwriters. 'Time's Up UK exists so no one has to say #MeToo again' is our slogan, and the fight for equality and against abuse and discrimination in the workplace continues.

While the international Time's Up movement focused at first on sexual harassment and bullying, in the wake of the Harvey Weinstein trial, the UK arm now focuses on insisting on 'safe, fair and dignified work for everyone', which segues nicely into the growing menopause movement. We need to call out ageism and sexism and the use of Non-Disclosure Agreements (NDAs) and payouts to 'disappear' menopausal women from the workplace, which makes no financial sense. Employers need to give women time and space to overcome or learn to live alongside their symptoms, and women themselves need to be better informed about the menopause and the benefits of HRT. Younger and older women need to band together at work to create a sisterhood stretching from periods to pregnancy to the perimenopause and menopause. Above all, the stigma and silence need to end. Time's Up for menopause discrimination in the workplace.

If anyone has pioneered talking about the menopause at work and in public, it is 68-year-old television executive Dorothy Byrne. When Byrne was head of news and current affairs at Channel 4, she gave the prestigious MacTaggart Lecture at the Edinburgh Television Festival in 2019 in the wake of the #MeToo movement, and courageously called out her own industry – which had 'no shortage of sexist bastards' – to cheers, laughter and occasional squirming silences. 'You know who you are – and so do I,' she told the men in the room. (She also admonished Boris Johnson for his reluctance to do serious interviews on television about his policies.) I know Byrne from the time our children were at primary school together – two Scottish mums often late to the gate – but I hadn't seen her for years until she turned up to give a talk at a Time's Up meeting following the MacTaggart sensation. She told me that when she'd given that lecture, she'd been on a huge, bloating dose of steroids to counter her giant cell arteritis, an inflammation of the arteries that can cause blindness if untreated. She'd ploughed on with her speech, undaunted, and took the TV industry to task about the menopause: 'The problem is barely discussed . . . often it coincides with parents falling sick and children taking major exams. That happened to me and life was a real struggle. Major broadcasters and larger companies need to take the lead by offering flexible and reduced working to older women so they are not lost to the industry.'

Byrne and I talked about the menopause, and eventually she commissioned (and generously shepherded) the menopause documentary. Later, I was having tea with Byrne and we started discussing estrogen. I'd dug up some interesting medical research on giant cell arteritis often manifesting post-menopause, due to estrogen deficiency. Byrne was feeling drained and exhausted anyway, so after our chat she decided to consult a menopause specialist about gradually beginning HRT. 'I wondered why I felt different, and I realised I was no longer waking up three times a night. (And I used to wake up thinking, *Broken sleep will give me cancer.*) I had much more energy and wanted to exercise more.' She has also lost half a stone, and looks incredibly well. Byrne's new job is president of Murray Edwards College at Cambridge (previously New Hall, but still a women's college), where she will no doubt foment revolution.

You can enjoy her MacTaggart lecture in full on YouTube,[28] but here's a highlight: 'Even getting your boss to understand there *is* such a thing as the menopause can be a problem. Kevin Lygo [Director of Television at ITV] is an inspirational leader but his knowledge of middle-aged women's medical matters is perhaps wanting. When he was my boss, we were meeting one day when he suddenly remarked that I looked seriously unwell. I said I was not ill. "But you've gone all red and you seem to have a fever," he said. I repeated, "I am not *ill*, Kevin," in what I thought was a meaningful way. He repeated that I was and I should go home. So I went back to my desk and announced I was leaving for the day. Everyone asked me why and I said,

"Because my boss has never heard of the menopause." More recently, Kevin has told me that this misunderstanding occurred because he assumed I was too young to be going through The Change of Life. What a charmer!'

Byrne's battle is proof that it's never too late to tackle the menopause, medically or culturally. The changes that are just starting in the workplace will make a huge difference to equality for women.

5

THE VAGINA AND SEX

I first met Stephanie Theobald at a reading of her book *Sex Drive: On the Road to a Pleasure Revolution*[1] at the Polari Literary Salon in London, which supports the work of LGBTQ+ writers and often provides a highly entertaining night out. Theobold was wearing a jumper and a delicate, gold, clitoris-shaped necklace, and was telling a rapt audience how she set off on a road trip across America in an orgasmic odyssey in search of her vanished sex drive. The joys of masturbating were central to her investigation. With ten other women, she attended a masturbation class in New York with the late Betty Dodson, the sex-positive feminist and author of the minor classic *Sex for One*.[2] '"Your left hand is your lover," the naked 85-year-old lady barks as she patrols the room with her own massive vibrator, which sounds like a cement mixer and resembles an old-fashioned kitchen device.' The audience snorted with laughter, and we had drinks afterwards.

This moment returned to me in all its glory when I was thinking about sex during and after the menopause, and reading yet another depressing survey in which 51 per cent of British women said that the menopause had adversely affected their sex lives, and around 40 per cent said they 'just didn't feel as sexy' since experiencing the menopause.[3] I couldn't agree less. Obviously, there are some people who take the gentle, sexless, pottering route after 50, liberated from the predatory gaze, and that's fair enough. They find new forms of sensuality and companionship. But a majority of women and their partners still want sex – which, unfortunately, can be painful for women due to changes during the menopause. The unwelcome hot flush can be a gatecrasher in many relationships. I have a menopausal friend in her fifties whose girlfriend is in her forties, and just as they seemed to be heading for bliss, the menopause got into bed between them. 'The problem is that I'm heading towards orgasm . . . and suddenly I get a huge hot flush,' my friend told me, laughing.

There are ways to give your sex life the second-half comeback it deserves, and orgasms, alone or accompanied, are good for you. They boost blood flow and the immune system as the rush of the pleasure hormone dopamine and the 'love' hormone oxytocin rebalances the stress hormone cortisol. They help with sleep, and sometimes with migraines.[4] They come highly recommended by Theobald, who is 55 years old, omnivorous and omnisexual, and has probably had more orgasms than anyone I know. I reckoned she would have some bracing words of advice for us on sex in later life, so I emailed her out of the blue. She replied: 'My thoughts would probably be linked to my topic of masturbation.' She was keen to have a chat: 'I'm now living in a cave in the Mojave Desert. (One year ago I didn't think I'd be writing that sentence in this lifetime.) But WhatsApp is good here.'

I called the cave. Theobald was on top form, and was hiding away writing a screenplay, the cool caves apparently part of a hippy commune, with Wi-Fi and running water installed. 'I was based in Los Angeles, and found this place in lockdown. In the seventies, this guy who looks like Moses built houses out of the rocks and there are amazing views and acres of pomegranate trees. The rattlesnakes I don't mind, but I'm scared of the spiders.' Now we had established the reason for temporary cave-dwelling, our cavewoman was full of useful insights. 'I've begun the menopause since we met. The hot flushes keep me warm in the cave at night. I've been masturbating a whole lot, and in came these cosmic orgasms. I have a lesbian friend in London who's found the menopause made her very horny.' Theobald said she also had female friends in San Francisco microdosing on testosterone to perk up their sex lives, but her main advice was to keep at it: 'You need to work out in the orgasm gym before you hit menopause. Make a date for yourself.'

There is a use it or lose it situation for the sporty 50-something to 90-something clitoris and vagina – keep the muscles fit and the juices flowing. Theobald is keen to advise the use of a good lubricant – more of which later – and regular masturbation if company is not available. Solitary sex sounds a little sad in English, but more fun in other languages. In her book, Theobald reveals that the Swedes 'threw a whole raft of Victorian prudery out of the window when their Swedish Association for Sexuality Education held a competition looking for a female-specific word for masturbation.'[5] The winner was *klittra*.

Theobald also talked about her heroine, Dodson, who thought 70 was the youth of old age and from 72 dated a 25-year-old man for a few years. Dodson's enthusiastic pursuit of sexual pleasure brought added rewards. 'It gives the lie to all that ridiculous propaganda about not sleeping and getting on HRT. Keep your sex drive up and the rest follows like jet fuel,' said Theobald. Certainly that gets blood flowing to the vulva, although the sex solution doesn't work for everyone's symptoms. But Theobald's enthusiasm is inspiring to us all; she is the Virginia Woolf of the vagina and says: 'All we need is a room of our own – to masturbate in.'

After talking to Theobald, I started to think about *The Vagina Monologues,* Eve Ensler's famous play conceived in the mid 1990s, and I read a fairly recent interview in which she explains her inspiration.[6] 'What compelled me to write *The Vagina Monologues* was curiosity. I was talking to a friend one day about menopause and she got on the subject of her vagina. She said it was dried up and prune-like and she didn't recognise it anymore. I was surprised to hear her, a feminist, talking with such contempt and disappointment about her vagina. I went home and starting thinking I have no idea what women think about their vulvas, labias or clitoris.'

After reading Ensler's interview, I was inspired to write a monologue on behalf of my own vagina as it hit the menopause: 'Congratulations on getting this far, Vagina! You're half a century old and still up for it. You've delivered three children whose heads felt like the size of watermelons, and pinged back into shape afterwards. You've provided regular and joyous entertainment in bed, and occasionally outdoors. You've even made it through an abortion. You've soldiered on through 420 heavy-going periods and over 6,000 tampons. And at last, with no risk of pregnancy and no pesky periods, you can relax and party. *Va-va-voom!*'

Except I had no idea, and not one of my contemporaries or older friends had told me, that the spongy delights and waterfalls of the vagina might start to dry up in the perimenopause and menopause. The estrogen that feeds the plump vulva disappears, the skin gets thinner and papery, and collagen and vaginal fluids reduce. What happens to your face happens to your fanny, and Olay doesn't make a restorative anti-wrinkle cream for it. Ordinary vaginal moisturiser is not always enough. The reason so many women lose interest in sex is often the sheer discomfort of a dry vagina and a shrinking clitoris, and not just their lowering testosterone levels or ageing partners. According to Dr Louise Newson, 80 per cent of menopausal women suffer from dry vulvas, but only 8 per cent receive help. Women struggle on, too embarrassed to divulge any discomfort. Shame, embarrassment, and cultural taboos remain a barrier to healthy sex, and most women have no idea there is an easy solution – roll up, roll up for topical vaginal estrogen, which could not be more simple or safe, since it is needed in tiny amounts and uses a different route from full-body HRT.[7] Topical estrogen comes in creams or gels you rub into the vulva area, or little pessaries you put in your vagina every few days. They release minuscule amounts of estrogen just to the area around the vulva, not the rest of the body, so they can even be used by some women who have had estrogen-receptor positive breast cancer.[8] Within a month or so, the estrogen will usually plump up the vulva, get the clitoris wagging and start the vagina self-lubricating again.

Vaginal estrogen is available on the NHS, and once you start, it's similar to moisturising your face and you can use it for life. Think of it as vaginal Chanel.

My own vagina seemed in good shape, because I was full of estrogen, thanks to HRT, but about five years after the menopause started I noticed I was getting a lot of unexplained cystitis and needed to pee more frequently – but when I took a test, it wasn't a urinary tract infection after all. I discovered, after reading yet another menopause guide, that the lining of your urinary tract and bladder thins too and can be helped by local estrogen in the vagina, or cream on the vulva, which suffuses the whole area. I called my GP to tell her what I'd found and she immediately prescribed topical estrogen, though she had never suggested it herself when I came in with a series of suspected UTIs. No one seems to be connecting the dots for menopausal women. The vaginal pessaries brought everything back to normal within a month, but I need to keep oiling the machine and taking topical estrogen for ever. So your urethra loves estrogen, too. The whole caboodle is now called genito-urinary syndrome of the menopause, or GSM, rather than the older term vaginal atrophy. Either way, it's as uncomfortable as it sounds – and it never need happen if women are informed and treated earlier.

Too many women get serial urinary tract infections and go back and forth to the GP, being prescribed antibiotics rather than vaginal estrogen. Everyone's chugging kefir and talking about the microbiome in the gut affecting health, but there's also a microbiome in the vagina. When estrogen is plentiful, welcome lactobacillus bacteria thrive on the vaginal walls and in vaginal fluids. It turns out that regular transdermal or oral

HRT can also increase the good bacteria in your vagina,[9] and it's probably a good idea to keep up the kefir and probiotics.

Dryness can even affect some transgender men who start enjoying the masculinising effects of testosterone, but retain their vagina and find that as estrogen levels fall, it gets uncomfortable. A year's worth of the tiny dose of estrogen that's in a pessary or cream is equivalent to a couple of HRT pills, so it doesn't affect the hormonal balance of the rest of the body.

We need a Great British Menopausal Vagina Conversation to sweep through midlife and older women so no one need suffer silently from a problem that can be easily and cheaply fixed. In the Channel 4 documentary I produced, we arranged for Davina McCall to talk with Helen Juffs, a therapist and reflexologist in Birmingham. McCall was fearless about publicly tackling the less-than-glamorous subject, and confessed that in the past she hadn't admitted to friends that she was on HRT. Now, however, prudery was over and vaginal estrogen was about to go from pubic to public on prime-time telly.

The conversation between McCall and Juffs took place in a yoga studio, often in the cobra position, though for a period of her life Juffs was in such pain that she had to give up yoga – and she was only in her forties. McCall, a heroic ambassador for lack of embarrassment, began: 'Vaginal atrophy – I hate that word. It sounds like your vagina has died . . .' Juffs explained what she'd been through. 'It started off with me being sore, and I kept getting cystitis, and it was really painful to go to the toilet. I sat on ice blocks for days and days. I just couldn't walk. I couldn't drive.'

McCall had similar experiences in her perimenopausal forties when she still had her periods, and had no idea what was happening. 'I had severe dryness, so severe that when I tried to wipe myself after I'd been to the loo I was having to kind of dab. I didn't know what that was. I had no idea that was part of being perimenopausal. We just need to talk about it and not be ashamed. It's something that happens to everyone.' Juffs agreed: 'One woman said to me, "I'd rather pluck my eyes out with a rusty spoon than tell my friends about this," which is awful, isn't it?' Juffs tried every over-the-counter remedy, from vaginal moisturiser to anti-thrush cream, until she got up the courage to mention it to the doctor, who prescribed vaginal estrogen. Now Juffs can do downward dog with ease. 'I did see a gynaecological specialist who said, "I think every woman should be sent a pack of vaginal estrogen on her forty-fifth birthday." So if doctors are saying that, it should be available on stands in the chemist!'

Although the NHS guidelines say vaginal estrogen is safe,[10] it's not available over the counter without a prescription. But Viagra, which helps men with their sex lives and has far more side effects, is in the window of Boots, the high-street chemist, from £10.99. My friend David, who regularly uses prescribed sildenafil (generic Viagra) says: 'It gives me flushed cheeks and watering eyes just after I take it, and often headaches and a bit of wooziness the morning after, but it's worth it.' Viagra is also a risk in combination with some heart disease medications. In contrast, vaginal estrogen's side effects are usually minor, occasionally causing vaginal itching or soreness.[11] Why are women treated so differently? Once again, it's Penis one, Vagina nil.

Even more ridiculously, the patient information leaflet in your packet of vaginal estrogen pessaries or creams remains the same as that for the old oral HRT, although, following pressure from menopause specialists, the Medicines and Healthcare products Regulatory Agency (MHRA) got round to updating the leaflet information on its website. But the old paper leaflets were still around over a year after the change in the advice: when I opened my box of vaginal estrogen, I still read terrifying warnings about clots, strokes and breast cancer, all of which are scientifically incorrect because they apply to a completely different product – oral, synthetic, combined HRT pills.[12] After exposing this, we gave the MHRA a right of reply in the menopause documentary, and it said the new leaflets would come through in time and that it was 'still considering the evidence on blood clots'. There is, in fact, a huge body of evidence showing vaginal estrogen does not cause blood clots.[13] Why is it all moving so slowly?

Dr Louise Newson, who has campaigned for years to have the incorrect advice changed, says: 'Many patients have told me they threw the pills or cream away once they got home and read the leaflets.' It's the same in America, where an editorial in the medical journal *Menopause* noted the positive effect physically, sexually and emotionally on women using vaginal estrogen and 'the deleterious effect of the boxed warning on women's health by discouraging clinician colleagues from prescribing, and women from using these highly effective low-dose vaginal estrogen products.'[14]

This failure to change the warnings for years is typical of the neglectful, lackadaisical, bureaucratic culture that surrounds so much of medicine for women going through the menopause. But guess what? Vaginal estrogen has been available over the counter in Finland since 1992[15] and can even be publicly advertised there, which possibly explains a lot about late-life Scandi sauna sex. The Finnish Vagidonna advertising[16] is bright pink and punchy, and shows fit women cycling, rowing and dancing. It's convenient, normal and free from embarrassment. Why can't we have the same here?

There is a growing public acknowledgement of the vaginal dryness problem (and the solution), evident in the hundreds of menopause support feeds on Instagram, Facebook and Twitter, the best of which are listed in this book's appendix, but its cause and potential treatment still remains a secret from older women not on social media or those who don't have English as a first language. Dr Nighat Arif gives menopause advice on TikTok to over 220,000 followers, and her video in Urdu on vaginal dryness has been a surprise hit, as she cheerily waves a diagram of the vulva: 'If you've had a very conservative Muslim upbringing, like me, you find that there's shame and embarrassment attached to talk about periods, gynaecological cancers and even breast cancer, and vaginal atrophy is definitely "under the veil" too.' She finds it hard to get the message across to older women, 'but younger South Asian women here are listening, and we can break those taboos and stigmas on TikTok. We can get through to the upcoming Gen X, and teenagers, who'll talk to their mums.'

Younger generations are not as prudish or embarrassed. I was alerted by my 25-year-old son to the Menopause Banshee character in the *Big Mouth* cartoon comedy on Netflix, in which teenage children navigating the craziness of puberty are followed around by Hormone Monsters, egging them on. The groundbreaking series is 'on a mission to defeat shame', say the creators. *Big Mouth* devoted an entire episode to periods, and in series three brought on the mom's own Hormone Monster, the Menopause Banshee, when she got a hot flush: 'Your womb is dry, like matzo meal!' cackled the Menopause Banshee. One of the creators, Jennifer Flackett, said: 'Women need to see those stories so they can tell those stories. It's in seeing it that you can also then say, "Wait a minute, that's not my story – let me tell you mine. Mine is this one." That's how you beget other stories.'[17] Aside from alerting the cartoon world to vaginal dryness, the Banshee is positive about the change and future freedom to come: 'This next chapter is yours to live, and now you have no fucks to give,' she says, cackling.

But what happens to the millions of women who know nothing about the Menopause Banshee or about the simple, safe, practical solution of vaginal estrogen and who may suffer years of agony, irritation and even permanent damage with more extreme injuries such as prolapsed wombs (the damage exacerbated by dryness years after childbirth) or fused labia as the whole vulval area atrophies? What about the women who can no longer ride a bike due to the pain, never mind have sex? Dr Paula Briggs is a consultant at Liverpool Women's NHS Foundation Trust, and she specialises in menopause and vulval clinics, and co-author of the textbook *Managing the Menopause*.[18] 'Vulvovaginal atrophy doesn't always start until a while after periods stop, so women don't associate it with menopause,' she told me. 'The link's not there in their heads.' My friend Janine had an apparently easy menopause, without hormone therapy, and says her vagina felt fine until she was 65, when it slowly began to get uncomfortable. She used non-hormonal lube and vaginal moisturisers, which were useful for sex in the short term, but they didn't deal with the long-term problem.

'My vagina was like a crisp packet,' she said, graphically. It was then that she headed to her GP for help, and got vaginal estrogen which solved the problem.

Dr Briggs added: 'So many women worry about avoiding cancer from HRT, but that doesn't happen with vaginal estrogen – this solution is a no-brainer, even for most women with breast cancers. Distribution uptake is a bit pockety for vaginal estrogen – if you're reasonably near an NHS menopause specialist, you might get it; otherwise it's random.' She says one upside of the Covid pandemic was that women have been much more candid during phone consultations. 'Women talk about not having had sex for two, three, four, five years, and it's worse after early or surgical menopause – no one discusses it.'

Atrophy of the vulva can be even more serious for women who experienced difficult births in the past that lead to episiotomies and scars re-emerging after the menopause. As estrogen declines, shrinkage of the tissue around the scarred, damaged areas of the vulva can cause pain and discomfort. Menopausal atrophy is particularly distressing for those who have suffered rape or female genital mutilation, bringing up past trauma. Psychological counselling along with the use of creams or pessaries is incredibly important for FGM survivors in menopause.[19]

Many women reach out for help only when their situation becomes unbearable, and then it is often too late for the body to respond to estrogen alone. For some really difficult cases of atrophy, Dr Briggs uses one of the new MonaLisa Touch lasers. Where the *Mona Lisa*'s enigmatic smile comes in, I'm not sure, but gentle laser therapy of this sort on the vagina stimulates a healing response that causes the production of new collagen, rehydrating and tightening the membrane lining of the vaginal wall. 'The laser works more quickly but probably has a similar effect to vaginal estrogen if this is used for long enough,' explains Dr Briggs. 'When things have gone too far, and nothing else has worked, the laser can work in a way that local estrogen cannot, but there's still a massive divide on the use of laser therapy.' So far there are no major studies on the long-term effect of lasers on the vagina, and the procedure is not usually available on the NHS, only privately.

Dr Briggs estimates that around 80 per cent of women eventually suffer from genito-urinary symptoms of the menopause, and believes we need to put this massive and massively under-reported problem in the spotlight: 'There's an expectation among women that they'll feel rubbish when they get older, so they don't complain when they should.' Joan is one of Dr Briggs's patients who did complain – six times, to GPs in Liverpool – and she bravely agreed to tell me her story. She was 50, working full-time and happily married, and explained to her doctor that she was struggling with painful sex. 'He told me I had a "hostile vagina"! I was actually starting to laugh. I was imagining my vagina looking evily up at me with a fag in its mouth. "Are you for real?" I asked him.' He sent Joan home with some lubricant.

Over the next four years, Joan went back again and again. 'I was feeling very heavy underneath, and I concluded I'd had some sort of prolapse of the vagina, but there was nothing there, just soreness. I wear a lot of trousers – I'm not a girl for skirts – and I was walking to the office printer when I felt a stab of pain underneath, and I thought, *Something's seriously wrong*.'

This time, she saw a young male doctor who suggested she

had thrush. Joan lost it and cried. Eventually, she was given an estrogen pessary. Around the same time, while in the bath, she found a that a strange, tubular fold of skin had appeared on her vulva. 'The doctor examined me and said it was just a membrane, but touching there felt like a red-hot poker.' She was itchy, too: like 'ants in my pants', she recalled. Sex was absolutely non-existent. Joan managed to be funny even about that. Her husband put on his reading glasses 'with his mobile phone like a miner's lamp' and had a look at the situation. Her vulva was different from previously. 'Neither of us is anatomically qualified, but we knew it was a mishmash and something had gone wrong.' Her husband was really caring. 'He said, "Sex isn't just sex. It's a whole host of things coming together, the joining of minds." It's the coming together, the emotional bond.'

But the discomfort continued for another year, and the small dose of vaginal estrogen seemed to have little effect. 'I felt I was whinging all the time. I was extremely frustrated. I saw young doctor after young doctor, and nobody knew what they were doing. None of them asked me to take my pants off, which would have been a start. I just didn't feel anyone was listening to me at all.' Was there an issue of embarrassment on both sides, or even doctors feeling that with older women some areas are 'out of bounds'? Thankfully, Joan spoke up again and was referred to Dr Briggs's clinic, where she discovered what was going on. 'My inner labia had got so dry they'd fused together.' Joan went on full-body HRT, and after a series of laser treatments, the labia were separated and her vagina started to work again. 'We could have gentle sex. I was cock-a-hoop.'

Dr Briggs is understandably frustrated by the lack of education and knowledge among GPs and women; every day she sees cases that have gone too far. 'I fully appreciate the challenges GPs face, having been one myself for years, but it's so important with urogenital atrophy to listen to the patient – and to examine them. We also need an objective method of diagnosis, and we're doing research on that now.'

The cost-benefit analysis of the use of vaginal estrogen is blindingly obvious, particularly in helping prevent the urinary tract infections that can affect around 20 per cent of older women, as well as other tissue damage, but NHS policymakers remain mysteriously unaware. Does no one think about women's well-being compared with the long-term costs of antidepressants and incontinence pads, or older patients who get sepsis after urinary tract infections and die?

My friend Jasmine, who featured in Chapter 4 and has worked for years in the ob-gyn outpatients' department in a big London hospital, told me what she sees every day: 'Prolapses. So many women in their fifties, sixties and seventies with prolapses.' Sometimes caused by multiple births, sometimes by obesity, and sometimes due to a lack of pelvic floor exercises, prolapses of the vagina can be helped by surgery, 'but mostly we push them back in and hold everything in place with a ring pessary and estrogen cream. The terrible thing is, it's not deemed an emergency.' Pelvic floor exercises are preventative, and so is estrogen to keep the skin and muscles supple. 'I can't bear the thought of all those women out there who aren't getting help,' Jasmine said.

It takes guts to get out there and shout about vaginas of a certain age, but Jane Lewis, a florist who gave up work in her late forties when mysterious vulva pain left her unable to stand all day, has been campaigning about this silence. After she worked out what was wrong, she became the author, with her daughter, of *My Menopausal Vagina*,[20] a self-help book with – appropriately enough – a multicoloured, rocket-shaped Zoom ice lolly on the cover. The book tells the story of Lewis's own atrophy; of chronic pain that so severe at one point that she couldn't even wear trousers. Lewis tried vaginal estrogen and it wasn't enough on its own, but she began to get relief when she started HRT too. She wants women to get a mirror out and get to know their own vulvas.

In her book, Lewis quotes a friend who is a carer in a nursing home. 'None of the elderly women are given estrogen,' Lewis learned from her friend. 'As far as she could tell, there's no provision for menopausal symptoms at all, other than the occasional blow-up cushion to ease the discomfort. It is truly horrifying to imagine the countless women the world over who are sitting alone in their rooms with unimaginable pain between their legs.'[21]

I thought about my own mother, once she mostly stopped walking and spent her days in a wheelchair, and how uncomfortable it must have been for her and many others with genito-urinary symptoms in her nursing home in Glasgow. But I hadn't heard of vaginal estrogen seven years ago when my mother was suffering. I wish I had. A survey in Sweden showed that one in six women over 80 years old was prescribed vaginal estrogen.[22] Yet again, we can learn from the Scandinavians.

If more women knew the science and spread the word, it would have a huge impact on older women's lives. There is a school of feminist thought that thinks estrogen supplementation is a terribly bad idea. Take Darcey Steinke, the author of *Flash Count Diary*, who said in one interview: 'I do think hormones have been sold to us as a way to stay young and keep your vagina pliable. It's almost like an Angela Carter short story. This very dark, medical, patriarchal world is feeding women as they age these drug hormones that will continue to make them sexually pliable.'[23] I'd like her to meet Joan from Liverpool. This isn't just about sex. It's about long-term health.

Exercising our vaginas is about health as well as pleasure, too. Those of us who have given birth know all about the pelvic floor, the group of muscles that hold up the vulva and anus like a trampoline. *The Pelvic Floor Bible*,[24] written by Jane Simpson, who runs a clinic for pelvic floor dysfunction, is a useful book on this. The strength of those muscles affects everything from continence to pleasure. There are so many women who can't jog or dance wildly without leaking a tiny bit, and during lockdown an article in the *Telegraph* by Saska Graville of the M-Powered menopause website revealed the existence of 'the "wild wee" network' for midlife women taking desperate measures in parks and streets to find a place to 'go' when public lavatories were closed due to Covid-19.[25] Pelvic Kegel exercises could come to the rescue.

When I was a foreign correspondent living in Paris and gave birth to the son who recently alerted me to the *Big Mouth* cartoon's Menopause Banshee, I went for a check-up with my *sage-femme* (midwife), the appropriately named Madame LeGaye at the Hôpital Franco-Brittanique. She always wore a perfect little suit and high heels with her white coat – I was in awe of her. She had a quick feel: 'You haven't been doing your pelvic floor exercises, Madame Muir!' I was like, 'It's two weeks since I gave birth and my mind and body are a sort of bouillabaisse.' She laughed and prescribed the usual French health service course of six classes of physio exercises to 're-educate the pelvic floor'. French women can also ask for sessions with a pulsing probe that exercises and tightens the vaginal muscles. Madame LeGaye added that every day I should pull my pelvic floor muscles up like an elevator for five stops, and let them down for four. 'But never completely let go,' she ordered. 'Hold that tension – and repeat!' For good measure, I was also given a leaflet explaining how to stop breastfeeding after six weeks so I could return to work – and probably to bed. Back then, the French were very keen to get mothers back into action – and lingerie – as soon as possible after childbirth. But the care and attention to pelvic detail was great – far better than my other births, in America (zilch) and England (a leaflet). I am still in awe of Madame LeGaye, and do my pelvic floor exercises when I'm waiting at the bus stop or on a really boring Zoom.

So, let's say you've got your entire vulva in tip-top working condition, and you're ready to go. But somehow you just settle for a bottle of pinot grigio and a tub of salted caramel ice cream on the sofa in front of Netflix, and think, *Unsex me here*, because your libido has completely disappeared. You don't even want to have orgasms with yourself. Well, yet again, hormonal help is at hand in the form of testosterone cream or gel, which can not only perk up your mind and energy, but your sex drive, too. Don't mention the mental benefits if you're asking your GP for testosterone along with your HRT, since testosterone is still supposed to be offered on the NHS only for problems with libido,[26] which can involve an official diagnosis of hypoactive sexual desire disorder (HSDD), a category of female sexual dysfunction. Once again, this harks back to hysteria rooted in the womb. I don't have HSDD – previously simply known as 'frigidity' – at all, and nor do many of the women who are prescribed testosterone as part of their HRT for all its other benefits. Regular women who just want to reboot their brains, perk up midlife sex and return to normal energy levels are unlikely to want to wear that shaming label of 'disorder' or 'dysfunction' and go begging to their doctor saying: 'Please, my libido is low.' Why is it that male medical supplementation with testosterone is about uplifting muscle, mojo and manliness, while female supplementation with the same hormone is about our sad, pathetic failure to feel desire? Hypoactive sexual desire disorder is not about women themselves, it's about their relationships with others, mostly men.

'That diagnosis is so fucking Victorian,' says Lauren Redfern, who is researching testosterone and menopause at the London School of Hygiene & Tropical Medicine. 'I'm so angry that women are given this label – 'You don't have a sex drive.' It pathologises women's lack of desire. Just compare the way we package Viagra for men with the language round testosterone for women. There are possible health risks for Viagra, yet it's available over the counter for men. For women there are *only* health benefits with testosterone, yet it's the other way around.' (By the way, sildenafil – the drug sold as Viagra – has nothing to do with testosterone. It started out being tested as a cardiovascular drug until researchers and joyous patients realised it increased blood flow to the penis.) 'If you look at men's and women's sexuality, women's sexuality is always connected to bearing children,' says Redfern. 'The sexuality of older women is not about bearing children, so it gets less attention, except when people make jokes about cougars or Mrs Robinson.' (Mrs Robinson was the 'older woman' character in the 1967 film *The Graduate*. She was played by Anne Bancroft, who was 35 at the time, opposite Dustin Hoffman, who was 29. I suppose the fact that film feels so outdated means cultural expectations do change, and at some point so will opinions on female testosterone. *Here's to your testosterone, Mrs Robinson!*)

While testosterone can disappear entirely after the menopause, for some women – myself included – the perimenopausal late forties were increasingly testosterone-fuelled, as the other hormones ebbed and flowed erratically. In her book *The Hot Topic*, and in various media articles, the journalist Christa d'Souza describes the perimenopause as 'the drink, as it were, in the last chance saloon"[27] and says untrammelled testosterone apparently means 'one really will mount the postman!"[28] D'Souza's group of friends, who were having similar unexpected spurts of lust before they hit 50, named themselves 'The 49-ers'.

On the Mumsnet website, there is a chat thread about women's experiences of the perimenopausal 'sex surge'.[29] One woman who'd had no sex for the last six years of her twelve-year marriage and had moved into the 'friends zone' with her husband, suddenly experienced perimenopausal mood swings and another 'pretty terrifying symptom, the massive increase in my libido – almost uncontrollable . . . Has anyone else experienced anything like this and come through the other side? It sounds like a good problem to have but I have nowhere to put these feelings and feel so desperate and scared that I'm going to do something life destroying. Any help would be appreciated.'

Soon there were 103 entries on the 'Perimenopausal "sex surge"' chat thread. 'I feel exactly the same,' said another Mumsnetter, who was 47 and perimenopausal. 'Been with my husband for thirty-two years and apart from when we were a lot younger I have had a very low libido. These last few weeks I've felt so horny it's untrue . . . hubby definitely not complaining. We've gone from once in a blue moon to at least five times a week! It's all I can think about! Just hope it lasts a while.' Other women said they had stumbled across the thread and one said it was a 'revelation, comfort and godsend' knowing they were not alone. 'I can confirm it is a thing,' said one. 'It's real and I have been experiencing it for about two and a half years now . . . The bad news is I too have developed a massive crush on a (married) male friend who I lust after with a passion. I know he fancies me and I am worried that one of these days I will take him up on the risky suggestion he made to me a few months ago.' The original post-writer summed it up: 'Somewhere on the internet a group of men are wondering where they can meet women like us.'

Psychoanalytic psychotherapist Jane Haberlin says the combination of testosterone dominance and erratic estrogen – which causes heightened desire – is part of the midlife earthquake that shakes up women and their relationships. 'There is that feeling that it's the last chance to reproduce. Before contraception was so widespread, there were many Downs syndrome children born from later-life pregnancies. There is that upswing, for some, of testosterone in the perimenopause, and later many women come into their own in their fifties, when kids have gone and men's testosterone levels are falling. When you're less maternal, you experience yourself more as a sexual being. You're wanting that affirmation and attention: *I've still got it*. You suddenly have the availability to have an affair; you're unfettered.'

These affairs are also thrillingly unpredictable, as women find their old patterns of sexual attraction changing in the perimenopause. I have two postmenopausal friends who left traditional marriages when they fell in love with women – late-life lesbians who have found a new direction not just between the sheets but in wider creative life. In *Married Women Who Love Women*, author Carren Strock says: 'I'd been married [to a man] for twenty-five years when I fell in love with my best friend, some years before I reached menopause.' Starting her first lesbian relationship, she concluded, 'Menopause is nature's way of releasing that excess baggage we've harboured for years . . . sometimes that baggage is so deeply embedded that we don't even realise we're carrying it until we begin our passage through perimenopause.'[30] Strock also mentions a trans man who had a surgically-induced menopause after cancer, and said: 'I was relieved because I never wanted those parts . . . Oddly, I did sort of notice my lesbianism and transness around that time.'[31]

Changing and reawakened desires may be joyous, but they are never simple: rebuilding a sex life that has collapsed during the menopause, or dealing with desire that has been reactivated by hormone replacement, is not easy for many patients, says Dr Louise Newson. 'Some women I see haven't had sex for years, so it can be daunting to go straight in with intercourse.' Of course, not everyone wants, or indeed needs, to have penetrative sex, and nor is rekindling desire about hormones alone. 'Others have no self-esteem, or have experienced a complete loss of self-worth during the menopause. Just holding a partner's hand and being spoken to can be a way of creating intimacy; people need to take back simple pleasures before going straight into wondering what position they should be in.'

Yet the menopause, with all its ups and downs and even new relationships, can also be a time to completely reboot and refresh your sex life. There's something about the honesty you have to find in yourself to navigate this difficult time that can also translate into a new kind of erotic intimacy with a long-term partner, or daring activities with a fresh one. You've nothing to hide now, you're comfortable in your own skin – although good lighting in the bedroom is always a plus.

So many people in midlife turn to mindfulness and meditation, and that's definitely worth continuing more actively beneath the sheets. Obviously, when I saw the book *Tantric Sex and Menopause*[32] advertised, I had to send for it, but I was disappointed: it is very much about soldiering on and making the best of things without hormones. Vaginal dryness and pain are common struggles to be borne, say the authors, and instead we should bring more awareness to our breasts. But why live with daily vaginal discomfort? It reminds me of the title of Jeanette Winterson's novel about her ultra-religious mother: *Why Be Happy When You Could Be Normal?* There is much more upbeat literature available on tantric sex, as well as practical couples' courses. That slow mind-body connection is mind-blowing, so it's worth a trawl through the 'tantric' and 'mindfulness' shelves of a good bookshop. My other later-life-love thought is 'Why Watch Porn When You Could Read Erotica?', and writer Rowan Pelling is always worth following for her juicy reviews of such books, from bodice-poppers to haute-literary bondage.[33] I'll leave you to google the best female-friendly pornography, but there's some very practical advice out there on websites like OMGyes,[34] which charges a one-off fee for access to a wide variety of real women's filmed experiences of self-caressing and orgasm, with some advice on thrilling new skills like 'hinting, layering, signalling and orbiting' – and then there's a tour of the 'G-regions'. All very tasteful and useful, and apparently Emma Watson recommends it. *Wingardium clitorosa!*

Finally, we end this tour of the nether regions with a visit to that den of iniquity, Royal Tunbridge Wells. There, among the tea shops, in a genteel terraced house, live Sam and Paul Evans, a lovely midlife couple who run the thriving Jo Divine[35] sex toy business, which caters to the mature client in particular. I went to visit them when we were filming with Davina McCall for the menopause documentary, and over their Cath Kidston tablecloth we learned of a secret world. Their oldest client is 95 and is still having orgasms with her collection of vibrators, and Jo Divine's new clitoral air-pulse toy has brought some women to orgasm for the first time ever in their fifties. I found that rather moving, but also sad.

Sam Evans, who is a former nurse, often chats with clients on the phone. She is a world expert on lube and believes there should be a tube of it in every woman's bedside drawer. 'Talking to clients, I often realise they need to look after their intimate health, with estrogen, a vaginal moisturiser and a good oil- or water-based lubricant – something plain. You don't need a lime-green vulva or glitter from your lubricant.

All those additives will only give you itching or thrush.' As she told me this, Evans was sitting on her sofa, wearing a nice patterned blouse, holding the biggest pink vibrator I have ever seen. Betty Dodson would have been proud. Then Evans showed us a small, unassuming purple clitoral stimulator which combined air-pulse wave technology with vibrations. McCall said: 'Oh my god! I've heard about those! My friend tried one and she said her legs shot out like a goat! *A goat! What does that even mean?*'

So who knows what delights lie ahead in the second half-century of your sex life? One of Dr Newson's patients, in her sixties, had a surprising turnaround after first coming into the consulting room in a terrible state, needing HRT and vaginal estrogen. It took a year for her to get back to normal but she saw results several months before then. 'She had a very supportive husband, and he came with her for her six-month check-up,' says Dr Newson. When the couple returned, they seemed very cheerful in the waiting room, if not a little frisky. 'They came into the consulting room and confessed: "We hadn't had sex for fifteen years – but we're having it now!"'

6

EARLY AND LATE MENOPAUSE

Harlow, Essex, 1994. Hayley Cockman was 13 years old and her favourite music was by East 17, a boy band from Walthamstow. She still had a denim jacket with another boy band – Bros – emblazoned on the back but she was moving on up. Shell suits were in fashion. Her favourite perfumes were The Body Shop's White Musk, and Anaïs Anaïs. She was ready to dive into teenage life at her school. She'd had her first period at 12. Then, less than a year later, they stopped for ever.

At 14, still with braces on her teeth, she started getting night sweats. 'I had to get up and change my nightie. I got a lot of hot flushes at school, and I couldn't concentrate on what was going on in lessons.' She didn't say a word to her girlfriends at school, but eventually told her mum, 'I feel weird.' They went to the GP, had a blood test, and she was sent to the gynaecologist for an ultrasound. 'They found I only had a small womb, one ovary and no eggs. They told me I had premature ovarian failure.' Cockman was in early menopause, now known as premature ovarian insufficiency, or POI, in which the ovaries stop producing normal levels of estrogen and may not produce eggs. The condition affects 1 in 100 women under 40, but very few as young as 14. POI is different from the menopause, however, as occasionally, either naturally or with top-up hormones, it can be reversed. 'I remember being in that hospital room and my mum was bawling her eyes out, and I was comforting her, asking her not to cry.'

Cockman is now 40 years old and married, but the meaning of that moment in 1995, after the ultrasound, is very different in retrospect. She still feels a quiet grief about the children she can never bear. 'The doctor just put me on HRT pills straight away, but what I didn't think about then was how much infertility would matter. All the doctor said was, "Well, it's not as if she would be trying to have a family anytime soon, anyway."' But when her friends started getting pregnant and saying, 'Isn't it about time you popped one out, Hayley?' she felt jealous and distraught. 'I would cope with it by doing manic exercise for a few weeks and stop, and then my mental health would suffer.'

Infertility and the menopause make a toxic double bill, but Cockman received no counselling and was then just left to go it alone, struggling with an oral HRT that wasn't really working for her. She went back and forth to the doctor with hot flushes, insomnia and hair loss, as the HRT dose wasn't high enough for a young woman. But the doctors didn't make the connection between these symptoms and a shortfall in her POI treatment, and were very dismissive. 'I think they thought I was some kind of hypochondriac.'

Dr Louise Newson says: 'Many GPs and gynaecologists have not been trained in the different hormone levels needed by younger women with POI – which is sometimes double or triple the dose of estrogen given to a postmenopausal woman, and they also need testosterone.' Hayley had no libido, which could have been in part due to low testosterone levels, but didn't dare tell anyone. Only now, 25 years later and after going to a private menopause specialist, has she been given the appropriate hormones. All of them are available on the NHS – but her GP didn't have the specialist knowledge to prescribe them. More education is needed, on the part of patient and doctor, in order to help younger women experiencing POI.

'When I say to people, "I went through menopause before my mum did," they're really shocked,' says Cockman. But in the last year, she has decided to talk in public about her experience. 'I've lived with it so long. It's something I've always hidden.' Cockman and her husband decided to try to adopt, and in autumn 2020 she started writing about their adoption journey on Instagram. The account (@prematuremenopause14) has also become a go-to resource for young women with POI today. 'Showing your own vulnerability can find you some amazing friends,' says Cockman. She is also planning to start giving talks in schools 'so girls can learn from a real-life experience'. They'll identify with the girl with braces who fancied the boy band from Walthamstow.

Premature ovarian insufficiency can run in families but is often rendered invisible because many younger women feel stigma, shame and embarrassment talking in public about it, and it is rarely seen in the media or given much space in the medical curriculum. But it is more common than most people realise, with 1 in 1,000 women experiencing the menopause under the age of 30, 1 in 100 under the age of 40 and 5 per cent of women aged 40–45.[1] While the 50-something hot-flush brigade can at least enjoy some camaraderie, earlier menopause is a lonely place. A POI diagnosis when you are even younger is very difficult to come to terms with, and women sometimes suffer anxiety, depression and grief over the loss of fertility.

When Cockman was diagnosed, there was nowhere for young women with POI to go. But in 1999, the national charity The Daisy Network[2] was launched by volunteers to create a support network for women with the condition, provide them with the latest information on HRT and discuss options for assisted conception. The website tackles the health issues and some sensitive emotional subjects, such as 'Handling a pregnancy announcement when you have POI' and 'Sister egg donation'. The charity also tries to raise awareness of POI among GPs and the broader medical community. One of the volunteer doctors answering women's questions in live sessions is Dr Rebecca Gibbs, a consultant obstetrician and gynaecologist who I happened to meet at my own check-up at the Royal Free Hospital in London. As a Black British woman, Dr Gibbs has helped change the face of early menopause – she realised a few years ago that every photograph on The Daisy Network's website was white, and with her encouragement it is now much more inclusive: 'When you're there in person at our annual Daisy Day, it's pleasantly diverse. There is also a group of young Black girls with POI on Facebook, and we're connecting up. There's so little for Black women, even on social media, about the menopause.' Scientific research is also lacking – there's almost nothing on the British Black or Asian menopause experience, and that needs to be rectified. In the USA, the Study of Women's Health Across the Nation (SWAN)[3] shows that Black American women tend to get more frequent and severe hot flushes and are more likely to get hysterectomies than white women. That means many Black women are entering menopause earlier and bearing those long-term health risks sooner. There's a growing conversation about 'allostatic load' and 'racial weathering',[4] in which poverty, stress and generations of racism add to health burdens, bringing about an earlier menopause – and shorter lives.[5]

Dr Gibbs's own realisation of unexpected hormonal changes began when she was 31. 'I discovered I had POI when my husband and I went for fertility treatment, and I started taking hormones to help with that and realised what had been missing all these years. I no longer had joint pain and exhaustion – and they had been difficult to manage in a career in obstetrics; difficult emotionally.' Her fertility treatment was unsuccessful, but it changed the way she came to practise gynaecology. 'It's so, so important that people get their hormones back. It changes your life. I didn't understand until then. As a gynaecologist, I'd have been more prone to dismiss symptoms like my own pain and exhaustion in women of my age or younger. But you're never too young to start hormones if you're suffering from POI. When you look at The Daisy Network, you see thousands of young women taking their HRT and leading happy, healthy, productive lives.'

Hormones move in mysterious ways – there one day, gone that next – but you certainly don't expect to see the words 'birth' and 'menopause' juxtaposed. Yet that's what happened to Emily Fisher. In the middle of the first Covid-19 lockdown, when most households were going batshit crazy anyway, Fisher had more reasons than most to desperately cling to her health and sanity: she was home alone with twin boys she'd just had by Caesarean section, was also looking after her three-year-old daughter, and her husband was working full-time as an A&E consultant. Then she discovered she was in full menopause – at the age of 29.

'I got in a bad state. I knew about the emotional roller-coaster after having a baby,' says Fisher, who had worked as an NHS mother-and-baby health visitor in Bristol, 'but this was different.' Fisher's mother had a premature menopause at 35, and Fisher had been diagnosed with POI at 25 and given a boost from a fertility drug to help her conceive the twins. 'When the twins were three months old, I started feeling terrible – much more exhausted than the first time. I was waking up at night, dripping with sweat, and my period came back so heavily I needed a tampon and a pad. I'd find the bed sodden when I had to get up to feed the boys. It was really, really hard,' Fisher says. 'I usually just deal with the physical stuff and get on with it, but when my mood started to get really low, I knew I needed help.'

During lockdown, Fisher struggled to get the recognition or treatment that she needed. After several unproductive phone consultations with her GP, she had to turn to the private doctor who had helped with her fertility, and was eventually put on HRT to increase her estrogen levels. 'In three days, I was a different person.' She explains the feeling: 'My eyes were stinging, looking out into the garden at the sunlight. I realised it was because I'd been seeing in black and white for so long.' Lockdown phone calls, rather than in-person consultations, often prevented doctors from picking up clues to patients' problems from their facial expressions and physical responses – so if it was hard for Fisher, a health professional, to get her point across over the phone, what can it have been like for women with disabilities or communication difficulties?

At the time I interviewed her, Fisher was planning to go back to work part-time after an incredibly tough year at home. 'I still don't feel a hundred per cent,' she told me, having suffered with further HRT problems, caused by progesterone intolerance. 'It was agony. The progesterone gave me so much bloating, my pregnancy hernias from the twins popped out again.' The progesterone also affected her mood. Progesterone or progestin intolerance affects a small percentage of women, but there are ways round it, often related to how the progesterone is taken, be that orally, or vaginally through a Mirena coil – an intrauterine device, or IUD, that releases small amounts of progestin directly into your womb, and is a form of contraception too. Unfortunately, waiting lists to have this kind of coil fitted on the NHS can be very long, and the cost of having one fitted privately is around £800.

Fisher's struggle was Sisyphean – not rolling a boulder up a hill for eternity, but endlessly carrying her big twin babies up and down the stairs, caring for her three children mostly on her own while her husband was on the hospital frontline. (And yet she had shiny hair and wore a smart jumper for our Zoom – I always found it hard enough to get just my three kids dressed when they were all under five, never mind myself. Respect.) Fisher is medically informed, articulate and knows the Bristol-area health system backwards, yet she was left struggling for almost a year, when a menopause specialist could have sorted her out straight away. Fisher also made a courageous decision to speak up publicly about her difficulties. 'Before this, I somehow felt ashamed about talking about my menopause when

I'm so young. Most of my friends didn't know.' But Fisher, like Hayley Cockman, decided to start an Instagram account, @motheringandthemenopause, which tells her story (and includes a gorgeous photo of the twins parcelled up together in a blanket). 'One of my male friends started following it. He was really sympathetic. He said, "Why didn't you tell us this before?"'

If the menopause is taboo, there's an extra layer of that stigma around POI for many women and the men around them, coupled with massive ignorance about how common the condition is. Cockman and Fisher both had very different experiences, but for anyone, when periods go missing for months, it is incredibly important to have your hormone levels tested and ask to be referred to a gynaecologist. Women who leave POI untreated, and live with hormone deficiency for decades, are much more at risk of Alzheimer's, dementia and heart disease,[6] as well as having to suffer menopause-like symptoms day-to-day.

Early menopause can also be caused by certain surgical procedures and cancer treatments, which can have different – and sometimes more sudden – effects than POI. Surgical menopause occurs when a woman has one or both of her ovaries removed (oophorectomy) or after a hysterectomy (the removal of the womb). Often both operations are done together. The removal of ovaries can be necessary to prevent ovarian or breast cancer related to the BRCA gene, to treat endometriosis and, as a last resort, to stop premenstrual dysphoric disorder (PMDD). Surgical menopause at any age has instant, nuclear effects, and women are rarely prepared for the sudden physical trauma post-operation and the long-term mental recalibration that follows. In the book *Surgical Menopause – Not Your Typical Menopause*,[7] menopause specialist Dr Jane Davis concurs: 'When I first started training in menopause, I was incredulous that women could have their ovaries taken away without really understanding the consequences.' So-called chemical menopause, meanwhile, can occur after chemotherapy, and radiotherapy treatment can also bring on symptoms of the menopause, but often women cannot at first differentiate these from the side effects of their treatment and may not realise that it is happening.

Any form of premature menopause – be it POI, surgical or chemical – can bring dangers, putting you at increased risk of osteoporosis, cardiovascular disease and cognitive impairment[8] if hormone replacement therapy is not used, and fortunately younger age groups are not at risk from breast cancer even from the less-healthy forms of HRT. Women under the age of 45 who have surgical menopause without hormone replacement are more likely to show early signs of Alzheimer's disease[9] than women who have a normal menopause, unless they take HRT, and they should also get checked for osteoporosis. Cockman went for her first DEXA bone scan in 2021, worried that she might have developed the bone density of a post-menopausal 76-year-old woman even though she is only 40, but the HRT had protected her: 'They said my bones were better than average – really strong.'

As well as physical symptoms, the cold-turkey withdrawal of surgical menopause can bring about huge psychological upheaval. Sometimes this can be unexpectedly severe, as in the case of psychotherapist and menopause counsellor Diane Danzebrink. She had a hysterectomy and oophorectomy when she was 45 to combat her endometriosis, and the sudden nature of her surgical menopause left her struggling with its impacts on her mental health. A keen horse rider, she refused HRT after the operation because she thought it was all made from horse urine (one brand of HRT, Premarin, is made from pregnant mare's urine, something we will come on to discuss in Chapter 8). But instead of coping as she'd expected, she floundered. 'There was this feeling of blackness and sheer helplessness. I was so anxious I couldn't leave the house, and my mum had to come when my husband was at work, because I couldn't bear to be alone. One day I found myself picking up my four Jack Russells and getting into the car. I drove to a dual carriageway.' It was almost an out-of-body experience, she says. 'I don't know how I got there, and I came about *that* close to putting my car in the path of a lorry. But my dog Henry started barking at that moment I was about to make the manoeuvre, and that was the only thing that stopped me. Essentially, he saved my life.'

Danzebrink went to her doctor and was prescribed estrogen (the kind made from yams rather than horse piss), started to feel better and decided to use her experience to set up a menopause support service.[10] She wrote about her experience in newspapers:[11] 'All those sleepless nights weren't wasted. I uncovered a world I knew nothing about: thousands of women online at all hours who, like me, were desperately searching for others who felt like they were going mad.' She discovered women out there of all ages, in early, surgical and normal menopause. 'But why were so many struggling? I made a promise to myself that if I ever felt like me again, I would find out what was going wrong and make sure I did something to change it.'

Danzebrink started the #MakeMenopauseMatter petition on Change.org to demand mandatory menopause training for all GPs, the provision of menopause guidance in every workplace, and for the menopause to be included in the new Relationships and Sex Education curriculum in secondary education – a battle she won in schools in 2019. Teenagers are now being taught that periods end, as well as begin.

The rate of surgical menopause is increasing around the world, with a creeping use of hysterectomy and oophorectomy as a surgical solution to 'women's problems' like heavy periods – rather than, perhaps, a carefully titrated use of body-identical hormones or a Mirena coil.[12] And often, when ordinary people say hysterectomy, they mean the loss of ovaries, too – half of women in the US lose both at once. There, one third of women have a hysterectomy before they are 50 – it costs $20,000 and is a nice, steady earner for the health industry. In Germany, the rate is even higher, and in the UK one in five women will have a hysterectomy, at a rate of 55,000 a year.[13] In India – and this shocking statistic merits a fuller investigation – the average age of hysterectomy is 34 years old.[14] It seems as soon as women have sufficiently reproduced, doctors are happy to rip out wombs and ovaries, which no longer serve a useful purpose – apart from, that is, keeping women healthy with a supply of hormones. This highlights the scant regard for women's health worldwide and the incredible ignorance of the role of hormones in long-term mental and physical health. Not looking after women's hormones following a hysterectomy is a dereliction of duty: in a study of 10,000 hysterectomised American women, HRT use decreased their risk of dying of heart disease and other illnesses by a third, compared with those on a placebo.[15] When I was on phone-in programmes on Irish RTÉ radio and BBC Scotland following the documentary with Davina McCall, dozens of women called in with the same story: they had a surgical menopause in their thirties or forties, and were left to cope alone. There was no proper follow-up, and many were not offered hormones at all, or told there was a risk of breast cancer from HRT when in fact it is tiny in the younger age group.[16] The suffering was huge – and unnecessary.

Of course, surgical menopause has quite a different meaning for trans men, as it is a positive step on the road to change, and most are already taking testosterone before the operation. To get a sense of the situation, I talked to Dr Vickie Pasterski, a gender-identity specialist, neuroendocrinologist and psychologist, who runs the Harley Street Gender Clinic in London, along with her assistant Dimitris Bibonas, a trans man who agreed to talk about his own experience. Dr Pasterski said menopause symptoms rarely come up as a difficult issue. 'Usually, replacement testosterone balances things out, so trans men don't have these symptoms, but that could change if people reduce hormones as they get older, or if they reach menopausal age and they've not opted for surgery. Each person is very different. It's difficult – patients are keen to be accepted for who they are and not have their integrity challenged. Many people don't want to keep their biological sex on their medical notes.' She added: 'We do need to pay more attention to long-term health outcomes in older patients, but there's so much attrition – people transition and want to move on, so we lose the chance to follow up.' In terms of scientific work, there's very little available on the trans menopause experience, but

I expect that will start to change. In the meantime, people mostly rely on internet support groups for information.

Bibonas, who is 23 and a science graduate, started transitioning five years ago. He first had chest surgery, then a hysterectomy and removal of the ovaries. 'I healed pretty fast. I had keyhole surgery and really no complications. No longer being in the wrong body is an enormous relief.' For Bibonas, the positive effects of his surgery outweighed the potential fears about early menopause: 'I didn't worry. I was excited about getting the surgery after waiting for years.' As it was, he had been on testosterone for so long that he had no symptoms after the surgery. His experience with hormones had started much earlier, in the summer he left sixth form at school, and he went to university the following term as a trans man. He has been on testosterone ever since. However, some trans men do experience serious symptoms after surgical menopause, yet research is almost non-existent and many patients find discussing the subject triggering. Bibonas is strongly aware that medical care needs to improve for the trans community. He hopes that 'as society progresses, people in the medical field will be more careful about the language they use – and a lot more educated.'

For those women still struggling with low-functioning ovaries, there is some hopeful new research. In a small study in China, injecting platelet-rich plasma and follicle-stimulating hormone directly into the ovaries helped restore ovarian function and periods for 11 out of 12 women, possibly allowing for pregnancy without donor eggs,[17] though Dr Stephanie Faubion, Medical Director of the North American Menopause Society, has responded with the reminder that: 'Additional studies involving large numbers of women are needed to determine whether this is truly a viable option for women with early menopause hoping to achieve pregnancy using their own eggs.'[18] Another option is the freezing of ovarian tissue, presently offered to some young cancer patients to preserve fertility before chemotherapy or radiotherapy. Keyhole surgery allows the removal of some ovarian tissue, which contains immature eggs. The tissue is thinly sliced and frozen at very low temperatures in a process known as cryopreservation, and years later can be surgically regrafted in an attempt to restore fertility. Some private companies like ProFam are offering this cryopreservation to delay the menopause. At present, though, the operation and storage is expensive, and there is limited research on how many years the grafts will work for.[19] But science is always moving forward. Will there come a time when the menopause is eliminated altogether, either by tissue grafts or long-term HRT?

While I was talking to Dr Rebecca Gibbs about the menopause in young women, she mentioned her oldest – and clearly one of her favourite – patients to me. 'She's ninety and she swims every day, summer and winter, in the Hampstead Ladies' Pond. She uses one pump of estrogen every other day – gives her some extra pep.' I was deeply impressed; sometimes the ice needs cracking on the Ladies' Pond, and my friend Deb and I have not yet managed to swim beyond October, despite our estrogen habits. But that remark led me to think about older women using and starting HRT if they feel the need. 'The best day to give up HRT is the day you die,' says Dr Louise Newson, who believes in lifelong replacement of missing hormones.

I was in Dr Newson's clinic, chairing a webinar for The Menopause Charity, when I happened to bump into Dr Newson's mother, Ann, who, though in her seventies, is still an examiner for the London Academy of Music and Dramatic Art (LAMDA); she also has a sharp wit and a predilection for dramatic scarves. It turned out Mrs Newson had been on HRT for more than three decades. 'I was in my forties, teaching drama students in London, and I just felt extremely tired. Everything was a real effort, and I also had three children to look after.' Mrs Newson's husband – 'the love of my life' – died when he was 40, and she became a single mum on antidepressants. But 'Mother's little helper' didn't help. 'It was a struggle to get out of bed, get dressed. I didn't think about menopause at all because I didn't get any hot flushes, and I'd seen my mother's friend get the sweats – horrendous. I went to see my doctor and he said, "You must be on The Change," as they did in those days, and sent me away.' Refusing to give up, she searched for a female doctor who immediately suggested HRT. 'I've been on it ever since and I'll stay on it for the rest of my life because I think it's the best thing since sliced bread.'

Did she consider giving up her HRT after the scare of the WHI breast cancer report in 2002? Her daughter told her not to panic, and Mrs Newson took a philosophical view. 'I've had so many good years, I've enjoyed life and I have no regrets whatsoever. I can't see the point of penalising oneself, refusing help, thinking *I'll get through that depression* and keeping going through eight years of hell. Personally, I've five friends who've all survived breast cancer and none of them were on HRT. I just think it's sad, talking to many women of my generation about what they went through, suffering at home. They had brain fog and got very depressed, and didn't have anyone to turn to.'

Mrs Newson has had two hip replacements – and temporarily got hot flushes when she came off HRT for a few weeks after the operation – but she doesn't have osteoporosis. 'The doctor said I have strong bones. I tripped in the garden recently and I was fine, apart from some cuts on my face, but they healed quickly.' She points out that she also doesn't have the thin, papery skin of some of her peers: 'I've got the crow's feet and the turkey neck, but my actual cheeks are not shrivelled like some of my friends',' she said, laughing. Mrs Newson's doctor told her she should stop taking HRT and she ignored him – some doctors still believe that HRT should be taken for the shortest possible time. 'We should have the right to choose. We shouldn't be told what we should do and life is for today.'

This seemed a rich seam, so I started asking other menopause campaigners about their mothers. It seems most kept calm and carried on, some took to Valium and gin, and some temporarily lost the plot. But wellness expert Liz Earle told me her mum was on HRT until she was 65. 'She loved it, but the doctor said, "Better stop now," so she did. She's now in her eighties, and a couple of doctors refused her HRT, but then one put her back on it. She said she didn't feel much different, "except I don't get up five times a night to spend a penny". Have you any idea what that sleep disturbance does to your brain? She's fit as a flea now.'

My friend Kirsty Lang mentioned that her mother, Patricia Hood, had been on HRT for about 25 years, so I fixed up a Zoom to talk to her. I first met Hood in Paris when she came over in practical super-grandma mode when Kirsty and I were both journalists juggling baby sons, and we all still have lunch together every year. To be honest, I thought the always-elegant Hood was about 75, but she said, 'Oh no, I'm 84.' She told me about her menopause: 'I was fifty and I felt like an over-strung violin and I was beastly to everyone. My gynaecologist said, "That's it, start HRT now and bypass all the menopausal symptoms." Then her fibroids (which can be fed by estrogen) got worse and she had an oophorectomy. Following this, she stayed on estrogen until the age of 75: 'I thought maybe by that time it had done all the good it can do. I still had a few hot flushes, but my energy was fine.'

Hood walks her dog for an hour every day, eats healthily and goes on rather adventurous holidays with her husband. 'I like riding in Argentina, and we've been to Antarctica three times,' she says, 'on a Russian icebreaker.' She said she became worried a bit about dementia (although she seemed to be firing on all possible cylinders when she talked to me), and after our interview she decided to go back on HRT: 'I don't feel any different but I hope what it's done to my organs will include the brain and keep dementia at bay.'

As we know by now, the menopause is not just a transition, but the hormonally deficient state we live in for the second half-century of our lives, and as Mrs Newson showed with her temporary bout of hot flushes, the symptoms don't always go away. In a fascinating study of a group of 85-year-old women in the Linköping municipality of Sweden, 16 per cent still experienced hot flushes during the day and night, and 7 per cent were still using hormone therapy.[20] There is a growing stream of research on older women who want to start hormone therapy a decade or more after the menopause and not in the 'window of opportunity' around the start of the menopause. Pioneering menopause specialists like Dr Newson in the UK and Dr Stephanie McClellan in the USA are trying a slow-drip method on older patients to get the body's estrogen receptors gently re-opening after years of starvation. 'Think of the soil being cracked and dry after a forest fire and imagine you add a deluge of water,' McClellan told me. 'It'll just run off. But what if you slowly add a few sprinkles of water, and then a little more as it soaks in? That's what we're doing with estrogen in older women.'[21]

So the picture for menopausal women from their teenage years to their nineties is far more hopeful than you might assume. While early, surgical and natural menopauses all bring their own difficulties, they have one thing in common: treatment is usually possible, and knowledge is key. Hopefully, the stories of the women – and the trans man – who have spoken out in this chapter will spawn more conversations, and the taboo will melt away.

7

ALTERNATIVE REMEDIES

'Are you suffering from Menopause Face?' asked a headline in the *Daily Mail.*[1] 'That's how one top expert describes the ravages hormones can wreak in midlife. Here she reveals how you can turn back time without HRT or Botox.'

I'm definitely suffering from Menopause Face, and it's purple with fury. Do we really need those negative headlines, particularly from a newspaper whose average reader is a 58-year-old woman? The statement doesn't even make sense – these 'ravages' (a laughter line or two) – are caused by a *lack* of hormones feeding estrogen receptors in the skin and facial bones. As for turning back time, it ain't gonna happen.

The headline accompanied excerpts from the book *Manage Your Menopause Naturally*[2] by Maryon Stewart, described by the newspaper as 'an expert on women's hormonal health' who has helped 'tens of thousands of women through menopause without resorting to the surgeon's knife or HRT'. Looking after your health in midlife matters, and there is certainly a place for the 'natural management' of the menopause, particularly if you cannot tolerate or don't want to take hormones, or just need an extra boost during the ups and downs of the perimenopause. The pressures of caring for everybody but yourself, from teenage children to ageing relatives, while also working full-time, can be seriously draining. And, unsurprisingly, your wider health and well-being will impact on how you experience the menopause; for instance, being overweight has been shown to cause more severe hot flushes,[3] so eating well, reducing alcohol intake,[4] and doing weight-bearing exercise[5] should be your top priorities, since those are medically proven winners in the battle against menopause symptoms.

We all know that healthy eating is important, and there are some foods, vitamins and probiotics that help more than others when it comes to the menopause; it's good to inform yourself on this. But why does that message have to appear in the media couched in ageism and unrealistic promises? 'You look in the mirror one day and, gulp, the first signs of a double chin stare back at you!' warned Stewart in the *Daily Mail*, and offered solutions: 'Add volume with oranges . . . eat oily fish for luscious lips . . . slim face with soy.' That's giving me a thrilling vision of sticking two oranges up my bra, ordering sushi from Deliveroo, squirting wee baggies of soy sauce on my face – and getting a *va-va-voom* body, a big fish-pout and cheekbones like geometry.

Actually, when you go into the book's detail rather than the silly headlines, Stewart's food advice makes some sense. The oranges seem to be vitamin C for hair volume, and soy contains isoflavones, which are plant-based phytoestrogens, weak relations of your own estrogen. (Phytoestrogens – more of which later – are some of the more promising compounds in the mad,

mad world of menopause supplements and solutions, which grows exponentially every day.) Women are flailing around looking for help – be it dietary, herbal or even spiritual – and the menopausal handbag is open for profitable business. Boots, the high-street chemist, told me online sales of its natural menopausal products went up 61 per cent in 2020 and Holland & Barrett said sales of its top four menopause products had gone up 28 per cent in the same year. According to one survey, 40 per cent of women experiment with supplements.[6] In this chapter, I'm going to look into herbal supplements as well as other popular and curious alternative remedies for menopause symptoms: daily ice-cold outdoor swimming, meditation, cognitive behavioural therapy, healing crystal rituals, and sticking a huge, purple, sparkly magnet in your pants. As we'll see, the benefits range from none to some.

First, let us take a trip to the menopause shelf of your local health shop to see what's available. Every overpriced packet and every Instagram and Facebook sales scam offers vulnerable, desperate women astonishing and astonishingly expensive cures for hot flushes, brain fog, weight gain, a dry vagina, mood swings, creaky joints – and, of course, 'Menopause Face'. Do any of the products make a real difference? I talked to the press offices at Holland & Barrett and Boots, and they said the top-selling menopause remedies on the high street are variously based on sage, black cohosh, soy isoflavones and red clover, mostly combined in tablets with names like Menolieve, Menopace and Menoforce. There's also St John's wort, ginseng, maca, sea buckthorn, ginkgo and evening primrose oil. While you're at it, you might as well load up with anything you're menopausally deficient in, including zinc, magnesium, iron, calcium, vitamin A, vitamins B12 and B6, and vitamin D3 (which is genuinely worthwhile for boosting the immune system, preventing osteoporosis and making up for a lack of sunshine). The result is an expensive shopping basket that most women cannot afford.

The jury on specialist supplements is still out and discombobulated. The evidence-based information on many of these menopause products is contradictory or completely lacking, and the quantities of each herb or vitamin may not be enough to have any useful effect. The 'THR' stamp, for a 'traditional herbal registration', means a product meets Medicines and Healthcare products Regulatory Authority standards for safety, but the fact that the ingredients are correct, with no additives, is not proof of efficacy, and regulations are much less stringent for herbal medicines than for conventional ones. Similarly, just because something is natural and plant-based does not mean it is without risks.

Take black cohosh, also known as black snakeroot, a plant-based ingredient that features in many of the top-selling menopause products at Boots. Maybe the wisdom of the crowds is telling us something that science does not? After all, black cohosh has been used by women as a traditional remedy for centuries. Under 'Complementary therapies' as alternatives to HRT, the NHS website says vaguely: 'There's evidence to suggest that some of these remedies, including black cohosh and St John's wort, may help reduce hot flushes, but many complementary therapies are not supported by scientific evidence.' While the research connecting black cohosh to the reduction of hot flushes is inconclusive, the research on the plant's risks is clear. At the time of writing, the Boots website states Menolieve black cohosh tablets 'may rarely cause liver problems'[7]. The Holland & Barrett website carries the same warning about its MenoCool black cohosh tablets: 'May rarely cause liver problems. If you become unwell (yellowing eyes/skin, nausea, vomiting, dark urine, abdominal pain, unusual tiredness) stop taking immediately and seek medical advice.'[8]

When I looked into the general academic research on black cohosh, this popped up: 'In recent years, products labelled as black cohosh have been implicated in many instances of clinically apparent, acute liver injury, some cases of which have been severe and led to emergency liver transplantation or death.'[9] Across the world there have been 83 cases of liver damage associated with the use of black cohosh, although it is possible that the toxins were also in additives to the herbal products.[10] One website, LiverTox,[11] reported the grim case of a 54-year-old American woman with no previous liver disease who took a liquid for menopause relief that included black cohosh, ground ivy, goldenseal and ginkgo. After three months, she got jaundice and stopped taking the product, but acute liver failure ensued and she died after a failed transplant. That's terrifying, and unlikely for most of us, but it proves it is always worth reading the small print on every natural, herbal product.

Doctors may not know the gritty detail, either – they have enough to do without becoming herbalists too. My friend Kirsty Lang went to her GP for alternative menopause relief after she had come through breast cancer, and he suggested black cohosh, despite the fact her medical notes showed she had previously had liver problems – and that guidelines from the National Institute for Health and Care Excellence (NICE) suggest it should be avoided after cancer. Lang researched black cohosh herself and decided to avoid it, and details her decision to return to using HRT after breast cancer in Chapter 10.

Some of the other ingredients found in herbal menopause products are much more encouraging. A meta-analysis of scientific papers on the effect of phytoestrogens (in isoflavones from soy or red clover) found that the products reduced the severity and number of hot flushes, even accounting for a placebo effect, and their safety profile is good.[12] You may not need to buy an expensive phytoestrogen supplement, however, since a few red clover tea bags or a bag of frozen soy edamame beans from your local supermarket will probably have the same effect,[13] with added fibre. A 2021 study in the journal *Menopause*[14] on 38 women found that giving a plant-based diet including half a cup of soy beans every day reduced hot flushes by 79 per cent. (Interestingly, the control group, who stuck to their normal diet in the 12-week trial, found their hot flushes went down by 49 per cent – a strange placebo effect.) The soy beans can be metabolized by gut bacteria into equol, a non-steroidal compound that seems to help alleviate hot flushes. What's not to like? Expect edamame sales to rise.

However, the amounts of phytoestrogens in these foods are tiny and studies have found they are better digested by Asian populations than by Westerners, due to differences in gut bacteria. Soy isoflavones can help in the rollercoaster stages of the perimenopause, which goes some way to explain why Japanese women, with their healthy soy-based diet, have a less miserable menopause and report fewer hot flushes.[15]

But are phytoestrogen supplements a risk if you have had

estrogen-receptor-positive breast cancer? The science is conflicted,[16] though Rebekah Brown, founder of the menopause supplement start-up MPowder, told me she was making a version of her new product with vitamins, minerals and herbal remedies but *without* phytoestrogens for women post-cancer. Carrie Longton, previously co-founder of Mumsnet and an MPowder angel investor, added: 'In the next twelve months, the team will be testing recipes for women who, like me, have had breast cancer and are therefore excluded from so many menopausal aids.'

The fact that Brown managed to raise over £500,000 in venture capital to launch her London-based company is a sign that the City knows this market is about to boom. 'We no longer have to explain that something that caters to fifty-one per cent of the population is not niche,' said Brown. The *Wall Street Journal* recently ran an article about all the new investment, headlined: 'Is the Menopause Product Boom Finally Here?'[17]

Brown was previously a researcher and brand planner, until her own perimenopause crash forced her to give up work and reassess her life and health, and what she saw in the menopause section in shops repulsed her: 'I felt I was in the end-of-life aisle. It reminded me of 1980s generic multivitamins.' She started doing her own research with a naturopath, herbalist and medical doctor and has come up with a bag of power comprising 24 plant-based ingredients including vitamins, minerals, soy isoflavones and Moldavian dragonhead, which sounds a bit *Game of Thrones* but apparently helps with skin health. One testing company asked Brown whether she wanted to include the 'clinical dose' or the 'marketing dose' of a product – the latter being the minimum amount you need to legally say the ingredient is in there. 'Lots of other supplements contain a lower, "marketing", dose, which is much less effective,' explained Brown.

She began by creating her Peri-Boost supplement, and her Meno-Boost includes the increasingly fashionable Indian ginseng or ashwagandha, which means 'smell of the horse'. 'Ashwagandha helps with hot flushes, anxiety, memory and mood. But it is important to source the right type – we work with Ashwagandha KSM66 which has a strong body of research behind it. There's also a bit of red clover in there.' For the Post-Boost product, after the menopause, they're researching various brain and memory boosters. 'There's a lot of interest in nootropics among young entrepreneurs in Silicon Valley, but I'm interested in the potential they offer us later in life,' Brown said. Nootropics are smart drugs and cognitive enhancers that claim to improve executive functions, memory and creativity. Who knows where the menopausal super-brain will eventually go . . .

There is a place for reliable vitamin, mineral and herbal supplements – but it's an expensive place. MPowders cost £69 a month. After I looked up MPowder, my Facebook and Instagram pages were taken over by an algorithm selling me all manner of midlife sorcery, offering a variety of potions, pills and formulas, often with a three-digit price tag. And yet those who can afford to will shell out. In a *Wall Street Journal* article on the growing market, Rochelle Weitzner, 51, who launched her menopause beauty company Pause Well-Aging after a hot flush, explained: 'It's a space that people are now starting to recognise as having a huge potential. There's a customer here, and this customer actually has more money than the younger customers that most [beauty brands] are focused on.'[18] Her 'accessible luxury' products include a hot-flush cooling mist for $39. You can also try a spray of cold water at home. It is easy to laugh at this, and yet we are all inexorably attracted to the words 'anti-ageing' and 'anti-wrinkle', when we should be pro healthy ageing instead. The midlife woman seems to exist to be fleeced, her disposable income and insecurity attracting stratospheric mark-ups on products. Her vulnerability is that it's easier to try to tackle exterior looks than interior mental and physical health.

One product that does seem to have a positive effect on the menopausal mind and body is CBD (cannabidiol) oil, which has seen huge growth in the supplements market. CBD is a non-addictive psychoactive chemical found in the cannabis plant – but without the THC (tetrahydrocannabinol) part that gets you high, so you can take CBD safely even when you're at work. Some studies show it has a relaxing effect, helping with anxiety, sleep and even joint pain.[19] More research is needed, but we know that CBD interacts with our natural endocannabinoid system, a collection of cell receptors, called cannabinoid receptors, in the brain, body and immune system. Hormones and endocannabinoids are known to interact with each other, and the lack of estrogen in the menopause seems to disrupt the endocannabinoid system. CBD helps boost it again.

Research into CBD's effects has increased since cannabis was legalised in parts of America and Canada, but the sample sizes are still small. Its effects on anxiety and sleep, whether related to the menopause or not, are particularly interesting. In one 2019 California study of 72 male and female adults complaining of anxiety or poor sleep, with various causes,

79 per cent reported that taking CBD daily decreased their anxiety for the whole of the three-month trial.[20] Sleep improved within the first month for 67 per cent of patients, but fluctuated over time. So CBD oil might be worth trying, particularly for women going through the perimenopause who often wake up at three in the morning filled with unspecified anxiety and panic caused by fluctuating hormones.

The amount of CBD used per day in the above trial ranged from 25mg and 175mg. That's worth noting, because while every chemist and alternative-therapy market stall seems to be selling CBD oil or capsules, it's tricky to check the potency. One study found that less than a third of CBD products actually contained what they said on the label.[21] Check websites and packaging to make sure products comply with Good Manufacturing Practice (GMP) standards and that the CBD has a batch number.

I talked to Jonathan Hartshorn, CEO of Dublin-based Satipharm, a high-end Canadian CBD company expanding into Europe. Satipharm has an ongoing tiny self-reported survey on the effect of its Gelpell capsules on perimenopausal and menopausal women that so far shows that 32 per cent saw improved sleep, 20 per cent an improvement in night sweats and 8 per cent an improvement in hot flushes.[22] Hartshorn is aware the data is only anecdotal, and said: 'We'd like to do more research, but there's been a significant resistance from GPs and menopause experts in treating a small number of patients with menopause symptoms to get an initial view of dosing and potential symptom alleviation.'

It is best to buy CBD oil in capsules from a reputable pharmacist, but the high street tends to sell products with very low potency – 10mg, when it seems from a round-up of research that larger doses work more effectively.[23] In fact, the UK Food Standards Agency has confirmed that anything less than 70mg per day of CBD is fine as a food supplement, although higher amounts have also been used safely under medical supervision for severe medical conditions such as epilepsy. There is interesting further reading on this in books such as Sarah Brewer's *CBD: The Essential Guide to Health and Wellness*.[24]

Less scientifically, I was keen to experiment with CBD oil on my friends and Satipharm sent over its strongest, 50mg Gelpell capsules. 'It makes sense to start the test at this high dose so we see a response early rather than slowly building up the daily dose over a number of weeks from 10mg,' said Hartshorn. I gave a month's supply of the 50mg CBD to my friend Vanora, feeling a bit like a drug dealer as I surreptitiously passed her the pack while we walked our dogs in the park. She is postmenopausal, has recently recovered from breast cancer and is on letrozole aromatase-inhibitors, which stop the production of estrogen.

A few weeks later, I asked how she'd got on. 'After about three or four nights on the capsules, I found I was sleeping much better, right through the night,' she said. But she felt the price, £140 a month for the CBD oil, was too much. My neighbour Karen also volunteered to test the CBD in her heretofore drug-free menopause: 'Overall, I do think it helped to reduce hot flushes. I was having about four or five a day, nights not so bad – just a couple, but enough to wake me. They stopped completely within a week to ten days of taking the capsules. I slept better. I stopped taking the CBD oil a few days ago and had a big hot flush this morning, the first one in about three weeks, and I also had one experience of racing heart and trembling hands, but it only lasted an hour or so and hasn't repeated.'

Because I was already on HRT and largely symptom-free, I didn't make a good guinea pig for testing CBD for menopausal use. However, I did try some of the smaller, 10mg capsules for a month, along with my usual HRT, and some muscle problems I'd been having while running disappeared, though I've no idea whether that was due to the anti-inflammatory properties of CBD or just because I was also stretching properly.

The sleep and relaxation effect of reliable CBD oil is worth considering for women who can afford it. In some states in America where cannabis is legal, the use of CBD and cannabis itself in the menopause is a huge trend. There are no statistics on this in the UK, but in the US, smoking cannabis joints seems to be helping with joint pain and other troubles – although vaping is the most popular technique. However, it should be noted that both those methods carry a health risk, and you don't necessarily know the potency. In the Midlife Women Veterans Health Survey[25] of 232 ex-military personnel in Northern California in 2020, an unexpectedly large number – 27 per cent – had used or were currently using cannabis to manage symptoms, and 10 more expressed an interest in trying the drug to manage menopause symptoms in the future. The average age was 55, and only 19 per cent of the sample were using HRT – clearly menopausal women were more comfortable visiting the cannabis dispensary than the doctor's office. 'This study highlights a somewhat alarming trend and the need for more research relative to the potential risks and benefits of cannabis use for the management of bothersome menopause symptoms,"[26] said Dr Stephanie Faubion, medical director of the North American Menopause Society, when the paper was announced.

For centuries, women have coped with the trials of midlife by getting stoned or drunk, and who would begrudge them that? But there's something depressing about the relabelling of chardonnay as 'Menopause Juice' in cartoons, or the marketing of a 'Menopause Mood Detector' novelty wine glass marked with three levels starting at the top with 'Don't Ask', then 'Bad Day', then 'Good Day' when the glass is almost empty. Alcohol is an instant reward, a de-stressor, a perfect solution for the time-poor, but often in midlife, just when you need it most, it turns against you.

When I was married, alcohol was a delight and a delineator of the end of the day, at early evening events after work, or at that buttock-de-clenching moment at 6 p.m. as we opened the cheap Rioja and cooked for the kids, before collapsing in front of the telly, half blootered, with the empty bottle. If you're a full-time parent with a full-time job, you don't exactly have time to wind down with an early evening candlelit bath, meditation or a yoga class, and so we seek other ways to calm down quickly. But I found, as many of us do, that our estrogen-deficient menopausal livers are less tolerant, enzymes are less able to break down alcohol, and red wine seems to trigger hot flushes – possibly through dilation of blood vessels.[27] What's more, as our bodies age, they lose water-volume, making it harder to dilute alcohol in our systems. In many midlife podcasts[28] and chatrooms, women are asking: 'Why is my hangover worse, when I'm drinking the same amount as usual?' There is much talk about 'grey-area drinking' – not out-and-out alcoholism, but a habit nonetheless. After being a solid, upright Scottish drinker for nearly four decades (I started early), always able to hold a few glasses and an argument together of an evening, I found in the menopause that I felt terrible the following morning after just two glasses of red wine: my sleep was atrocious, with unnamed guilt and anxiety percolating at 3 a.m., and alcohol's depressant effect wafting around for hours after I woke. Even though I didn't drink heavily, I needed a particular short, sharp running circuit that I named 'The Hangover Recovery Route'.

Luckily, I fell in love in my fifties with a man who didn't drink. After we'd been together for about a week, I thought, 'I want to be on his planet. I don't want to be on a different planet.' So I gave up alcohol completely on 1 January 2019 – and, to my surprise, it was just fine. It took a couple of weeks to get used to it, but every time I felt a mild 6 p.m. craving, I noted the fact I felt perkier and more energetic every morning, my skin had improved, any spots had disappeared and my eye bags had gone from extra-large to medium. You can't buy that in a jar. I still do cocktail hour, but with Fever Tree pink tonic, just for the ritual, and the dog now gets more long summer-evening walks.

While the solution to certain menopausal problems might be obvious, in terms of cutting down on alcohol and increasing exercise and self-care, we all know how hard those changes can actually be. The instant, dream cure is so much more enticing – which is perhaps why three quarters of a million women have now bought the LadyCare Plus menopause magnet, which costs £39. This powerful, teardrop-shaped magnet is encased in sparkly purple plastic about the size of a 50p; this and a smaller, round magnet clamp together either side of the front of your pants, four inches below your navel, and you wear them day and night. Magnetic therapy has been around for centuries, and despite negligible scientific evidence, we keep returning to it. The LadyCare website is most entertaining, and even includes a feature that asks: 'Can a woman have an orgasm after menopause?'[29]

I had an enlightening phone chat with Derek Raymond Price, the founder of LadyCare, who first tested the power of magnetism on his lame dog, by putting a magnet in its collar. Lo and behold, the dog was racing round the yard ten days later. 'The most important thing to remember is every lady's different,' said Price, explaining his revolutionary breakthrough. 'Some find the magnet works in the first few days but that's quite rare, but we see results in three months. The magnets are good for policewomen – when they're menopausal they take them off active duty with guns.' I replied, 'Do they really?' while doodling a little policewoman in my notebook with the words 'I'm Packin' Heat!' on her T-shirt. Price explained that 'declining hormones cause imbalance of the autonomic nervous system, which controls your body temperature, and for seventy-one per cent the LadyCare magnet will rebalance this.' This statistic is not from an independent survey based on rigorous research; in fact, the Advertising Standards Authority ruled against LadyCare in 2019 after a complaint: 'We told LadyCare Menopause Ltd not to make efficacy claims about their device in relation to relieving symptoms of the menopause, in the absence of adequate evidence. We also told them not to state or imply that the product had an established physiological effect on the body.'[30]

Despite the ASA ruling, ladies are still rushing to buy LadyCares like climacteric lemmings, undeterred by reports on Gransnet of a shopper being pinned to a Tesco trolley by her magnet, and a diner attacked at crotch level by cutlery on a hotel table.[31] I needed to know about the magnet's powers for myself, and Price kindly popped a few complimentary LadyCares in the post for me to test on my menopausal girlfriends, who were getting increasingly keen on being guinea pigs during the boredom of lockdown. After a few weeks of having the LadyCare in her undergarments, my friend Kate in Scotland reported back: 'Brain still damn woolly, but I've been much friskier than I was this time last year. One thing I noticed – my watch has gone mad! Could that be the magnet? No attacks of killer trolleys yet or space debris, but I'm keeping alert.'

I texted Portia, who is an American in London, to ask how her LadyCare home trial was going. You should know that her husband had metal braces on his teeth at the time. She replied: 'My pussy magnet? It's jolly fine. We had a cautionary moment when my husband approached but swayed away before my magnetic field clamped him to my pants. It's also wonderful to remove the device before a shower and watch the two sides clasp together mid-air and land on the bed like part of a Marvel franchise costume. In short, its genius is that I barely feel it, day and night. Excellent design. But it's made fuck-all impact in the two weeks or so that it's been installed. Nevertheless, I have grown fond of its magnetic, sparkly, purple presence. And I can imagine that a tribe of Mooncup millennials could become quite attached.'

But it's not millennials who are buying this woo-woo stuff – it's sensible, middle-aged women who are raising children, caring for ageing parents and working. Yet they are so desperate to keep going that a strange gullibility overtakes them. It doesn't help that the magical thinking often runs alongside serious medical and health advice. Take the website of The Marion Gluck Clinic in London which sells women 'bioidentical' hormones prescribed by qualified doctors yet also includes advice to 'Raise the vibration with crystals', in an article by Dr Vera Martins.[32] 'Crystals are great tools, gifts from the earth, that help balance the energetic vibration of spaces and people,' she writes, advising menopausal women to mitigate the nasty electromagnetic forces emanating from their phones, laptops and Wi-Fi with black tourmaline crystals. 'Get yourself a beautiful black tourmaline and place it on your desk close to you. Boost the space vibration even further by getting a clear quartz crystal for mental clarity, focus and positive thinking.' Some months after reading this, I interviewed Dr Martins, who is a naturopathic herbalist. I asked her about quackery in the herbal world and whether the crystals actually raised her vibrations, and she laughed a bit and said, 'That one I'll give to you!' But she did have some sensible advice: 'Herbal medicine should not be taken lightly. We are using active ingredients and there should be more awareness that a lot of products are really bad quality. The purity of ingredients is key.'

Dr Martins is not against HRT, but says that nutrition, vitamins, minerals and herbs can all provide the extra help we need, particularly in the perimenopause years, before some women turn to hormone replacement. Stress, lowered immunity, digestive troubles, sleeplessness and hormone imbalance are typical difficulties in the women she sees. She makes preparations tailored to each patient's needs – say, lemonbalm for insomnia, black cohosh or sage tea for hot flushes, as well as magnesium, vitamin D and omega 3 oil. 'I've seen very beautiful things happen in the clinic,' she said. 'I invite women to reassess the negative connotations of menopause, and re-invent themselves. The beautiful side of the menopause is that we slow down and listen to our bodies.'

I love the idea of the menopause as a time to pause and reboot – mine has been exactly that, and not just thanks to hormones. But when I looked up the menopause on the wellness section of Gywneth Paltrow's Goop website, I realised we were, in fact, consciously uncoupling from our hormones. 'Don't call it menopause: embracing the change,' says a headline on the site, and Paltrow gives us her philosophy in an interview in *Vogue*:[33] 'I think menopause gets a really bad rap and needs a bit of a rebranding. I don't think we have in our society a great example of an aspirational menopausal woman.' I snorted at that. Luckily, Paltrow is now 49 and ready to be an aspirational example to all, selling her Madame Ovary supplements for women at $90 a month.

Who do you trust in this world of wild claims and promises? I got an insider point of view from Liz Earle, who was given an MBE for services to the beauty industry over 20 years ago but has not been connected to her eponymous beauty brand for many years, returning to writing books and researching all areas of well-being. Her well-informed podcasts often feature scientists taking down false claims about herbal and beauty products, diets and health, and she is also the author of the informative books *The Good Menopause Guide*[34] and *The*

Truth About HRT,[35] among others. Of the menopause-milking industry she says: 'It is an endless path to hell paved with good intentions. Lots of people are being taken in by strange supplements, by quartz crystals that are supposed to make you feel so much better. Quite how have we allowed this to happen?' The minor improvements from herbal remedies and supplements are fine, and may work to combat symptoms, but is less likely that they will tackle the root cause of the hormone deficit. 'We spend so much money on "alternatives" when HRT clearly works better for most women,' says Earle. 'Women throw money at "natural" remedies which are more unnatural than replacing missing hormones with body-identical ones. We need to call out the charlatans profiteering.'

Dr Stephanie Faubion of the North American Menopause Society says no herbal remedy has ever been proven to work in any significant way.[36][37] There are, however, other routes that do not involve ingesting anything at all. Faubion suggests that cognitive behavioural therapy (CBT) often helps by reducing anxiety, which can in turn make hot flushes more manageable. CBT focuses on the links between physical symptoms, thoughts, feelings and behaviour. The very stress of an approaching hot flush can make the flush itself worse, and CBT can change the way we think about symptoms, and therefore the intensity of bodily reactions.[38] CBT is offered by the NHS, but the waiting list for treatment can be a year or more.

However, you can start meditation and mindfulness for free straightaway, even for ten minutes a day. Meditation is hugely helpful on the sleep and stress front, and there are plenty of apps, such as Headspace and Calm, that make starting the process simple. But being in a communal space and sharing the menopause and meditation experience with other women can amplify the effects. I interviewed meditation coach Lucia van der Drift after she launched her six-week Mindfulness for Menopause class for NHS staff at the Royal Free Hospital in London. 'I wanted to help people in caring positions who were giving so much every day but not being supported themselves,' van der Drift told me. 'Research shows even doing a week of mindfulness can make a difference to levels of anxiety, stress and insomnia. It produces emotional resilience.' Apart from mindfulness exercises like a 20-minute body scan, van der Drift also gave the women homework – just to breathe while waiting for kettle to boil, connect to the soles of their feet and take a few minutes of being still. 'In the group, women could talk safely about hot flushes or worries about cognitive decline and bond over that. I also tried to encourage a more positive mindset, getting them to write down what they wanted to do after the menopause change to build a sustainable life in the future.'

Therese Witham, a 53-year-old community midwifery matron who oversees more than a hundred midwives in the Hampstead, Barnet and Edgware areas of London, attended van der Drift's mindfulness class. 'I've got a big job with challenging patients, and I've got challenging teenagers at home,' explains Witham. 'At work I was feeling really angry, really furious, and that was completely alien to me. It was at the end of what I could bear, and anger is not the response. I felt I could just smash something. I needed a punchbag at work.' Witham's job also involves making public presentations about progressing midwifery, and suddenly she felt self-doubt and a lack of confidence. 'Logically, I knew this isn't the way I would behave but the emotion was overwhelming.' Mindfulness for Menopause was right on her doorstep, at 5.30 p.m. after work. 'It really helps, discussing with the community of other women, not being alone, because you feel if you make excuses in public you're weak. I don't think I would have been able to do it otherwise.'

The mindfulness was helpful in several respects. 'Lucia explained how your brain is affected, what hormones do, and knowing the technical stuff really helped me,' Witham says. 'I thought I was mad, and then this all fitted into place, and there were logical solutions. The second session was a real breakthrough in terms of symptoms – this heavy weight on my chest lifted as I breathed into the area and focused on it. The body scan released tension and the discomfort was gone! It was transformational at the time, and I'll continue to use it.'

The communality of meditating or just talking about midlife can make more difference than a Holland & Barrett basket of herbal remedies. The more women know and understand what's happening to them, the easier it is to handle; and the more women confess their struggle in the public eye, the better for all of us. Among the increasing number of celebrities speaking out is the television presenter Trisha Goddard. I met her at a #Pausitivity event – a campaign encouraging every doctor's surgery to display a downloadable menopause poster – that was organised by Carolyn Harris MP. Goddard, 63, had just been training for the TV series *Dancing on Ice* and was wearing a tight black jumper and a blue mini-kilt with matching tartan leggings. This was not a woman crushed by The Change. Goddard's menopause was kicked off early by chemo and radiotherapy for successful breast cancer treatment when she was 48: 'It was like being thrown at a wall. I went from zero to sixty with all the symptoms.' But she worked her way through the difficulties without HRT – due to the cancer risk – and exercised and weight-trained to keep her bones and body strong. 'I made my own luck,' she says. She found that red clover tea helped a bit with the hot flushes (so, I suspect, did *Dancing on Ice*), and she runs five kilometres every day, if not more. And alongside these lifestyle changes, she has one other piece of advice: 'Be selfish,' she says. 'Look after yourself.'

Exercise, from yoga to running to Pilates can also be meditative in its own way, and I have even been trying 5Rhythms[39] dancing at my blacked-out local school gym, which is like being in a club in Ibiza without the drugs. But the new craze for many menopausal women turns out to be swimming in ice-cold water. My friend Lorraine Candy, the former *Sunday Times* 'Style' section editor, who now makes the podcast *Postcards from Midlife*, is an obsessive cold-water swimmer. She can be found doing lengths in London's Parliament Hill Lido all winter without a wetsuit, and also swims in local lakes and reservoirs. 'I still gasp when I get in, but soon my skin tingles and the high just after I'm out is extraordinary.' The community of women also makes a difference – I have a friend who breaks a north-west passage through the winter ice for a communal swim throughout the year in the White Loch near Glasgow. The splendidly named Bluetits open-water swimmers have a 16,000-follower Facebook group and chapters from Pembrokeshire to the Essex coast.

Candy explains that the appeal isn't just the exhilaration, but long-term health benefits. 'The theory is that the shock of cold, particularly on your face, prompts a fight-or-flight response in the body, and the more we get used to that, the better, as it protects the immune system.' In a review of literature on cold-water swimming, Professor Michael Tipton of the Extreme Environments Laboratories at Portsmouth University noted that the stress and inflammatory responses of adapted cold-water swimmers were found to be lower than those of unadapted swimmers, and the regular cold-water swimmers also had increased concentrations of dopamine and serotonin, which produce the after-swim high.[40] It seems that cold-water swimming activates endorphins[41] and helps to boost your white blood cell count when the body is forced to react to changing conditions.[42] Over time, your body becomes better at activating its defences.

The winter swimmers at Parliament Hill Lido have become a key element in ongoing research into a 'cold-shock' protein found in their blood, which is being studied by the Department of Clinical Neurosciences at Cambridge University. Researchers have found that all of the swimmers become hypothermic, with core temperatures as low as 34°C, and in mice that cold-shock protein has been shown to slow the onset of dementia and even repair damage caused by the disease.[43] Professor Giovanna Mallucci, of the UK Dementia Research Institute's Centre at Cambridge, believes the discovery could point towards new drug treatments to prevent dementia.[44] She was fascinated that brain connections are lost by hibernating animals, like bears and hedgehogs, when some synapses die off as their bodies preserve resources for winter, but when they awake in the spring, those connections are miraculously reformed. The cold-shock protein could be the key to the formation of new connections. This may also be incredibly good news for the menopausal brain, although becoming hypothermic can be dangerous, particularly combined with other health conditions, so take medical advice and train up before your plunge. If icy ponds are not your thing, a cold shower long enough to cool your core may be helpful. One study showed that people finishing a daily shower with a 30-second blast of cold water reduced their sick days at work by almost a third.[45] Just try not to scream.

What has come out of all this research – once we discard the fanny magnets and fanciful potions – is that the menopause should be the fulcrum tipping you into a new way of life. There's not a binary decision to be made – to either take hormones or try alternatives. They can be complementary. The research into these areas is just beginning, and new options will emerge over the next decade. In the meantime, how can you possibly go wrong with an icy swim tanked up on CBD oil, followed by a mass menopausal meditation? It's about celebrating exuberance, not erasing wrinkles. Our long-term plan should be to replace the sad 'Menopause Face' with an ear-to-ear grin.

8

WHY IS IT SO HARD TO GET HRT?

As Ernest Hemingway once said: 'Remember, everything is right until it's wrong. You'll know when it's wrong.' This is very much true of the scientific rollercoaster of menopausal therapy. (I should also flag here that we will hear Hemingway's muscular views on the writer Gertrude Stein's menopause later.) We must acknowledge new research and question the old – if we didn't, we would still be using Victorian menopause cures: mesmerism, sedatives, opium, a large belladonna plaster placed on the stomach or injections to the vagina with a solution of acetate of lead, as well as improved 'moral management'. And, lest we forget, leeches on the cervix.

We need to move on, and think in an entirely fresh way about how we treat the menopause. This is particularly true of hormone replacement therapy, or HRT.

Some women may motor smoothly through the menopause, but 90 per cent suffer symptoms, some of which are utterly debilitating. The smooth operators are the few that produce an alternative source of hormones – testosterone in their adrenal glands or estrogen in their fat cells – to keep them going after their ovaries cease to produce hormones. But most of us find our back-up hormonal generator isn't working properly and need a way to replace the hormones that are essential for the smooth running of both body and mind. This book contains the latest research and opinions from menopause experts, but obviously, women should always consult a health professional about their specific needs. It's worth knowing though, that the British Menopause Society has said in its Women's Health Concern information that for the majority of women who can take HRT, the benefits outweigh the risks.[1]

Replacing your natural hormones is incredibly good for your long-term health as well as for treating short-term symptoms like brain fog and hot flushes. If you are feeling exhausted and demotivated during the menopause, lifestyle changes are not so easy. It might be a struggle just to leave the house, or to abandon the ready meals in the microwave or give up the half-bottle of wine drunk every night as a consolation for life falling apart. Instead, for many, HRT can be the first stepping stone to recovery.

Aside from the short-term benefits of HRT, the long-term ones are nothing short of astounding, but a lack of joined-up thinking on women's medicine, which remains trapped in a silo of sexism, means that those in charge of health policy do not seriously consider the fact that the transdermal estrogen given in HRT reduces the risk of stroke,[2] heart disease,[3] osteoporosis,[4] colon cancer[5] and type-2 diabetes,[6] and even helps with joint pain and arthritis.[7] 'The protective effects on health are extraordinary,' says menopause specialist Dr Louise

Newson, who takes plant-based, body-identical hormones herself and intends to stay on them for the rest of her life. She told me about a patient who arrived for her first consultation using a stick, limping up to her office, in agony from joint pain. 'Three months later, the woman returned and ran up the stairs.' It's like Lourdes, sometimes, in Newson's clinic in Stratford-upon-Avon. Despite such miracles, there seems to be no interest from big pharmaceutical companies, or anyone for that matter, in funding more research on body-identical HRT. That's because hormones in their pure form are not legally patentable, since they are 'products of nature'; if they were, you can bet that Big Pharma would be selling transdermal estrogen for billions, as 'The Elixir of Youth'.

But it's hard to have foresight about heart attacks, stiff joints and hip replacements if you feel not-too-bad in your forties or fifties. Why not just carry on delicately declining as nature intended? Osteoporosis may be invisible, but watching collagen in your skin decline by about 2 per cent a year after the menopause is salutary, as is the discovery that estrogen plumps it right back up again. It's the best and simplest skincare regime on earth. You still get wrinkles, but they're not so deep, and the bones in your face remain strong, avoiding a receding chin and sunken eye sockets. The real clincher for some may be that hormone replacement will stop you getting a 'menopot'. I only recently learned this ridiculous word, which refers to the pot belly women tend to get after the menopause and find so hard to shift. And a menopot often arrives accompanied by a muffin top. (Why are we so unforgiving about our own bodies? And why do we use cookery terms?) But excess fat round the middle is dangerous, as we have seen only too recently, with obese or overweight people making up 62 per cent of Covid-19 deaths.[8]

But the good news is that a Swiss study of 1,500 postmenopausal women showed that those on HRT had much lower levels of dangerous fat – deep in the abdomen, around the internal organs – than those who were not on HRT.[9] That deep fatty tissue makes tiny amounts of a postmenopausal estrogen called estrone, while your body actually craves the more powerful premenopausal estrogen, estradiol, instead. Abdominal obesity is associated with metabolic syndrome – diabetes, blood pressure and obesity, all risk factors for cardiovascular disease – and HRT helps prevent that. In the study, hormone users had a slightly lower body mass index (BMI) too. Of course, there is also the 'healthy-user bias': women who get themselves onto HRT tend to be healthier and wealthier in the first place. We need to change that, and to get the message out to more women, particularly those at risk of the diabetes and obesity epidemics.

We need to question the conventional wisdom, which says that HRT causes breast cancer and that the risks of taking HRT outweigh the benefits. What most people – including me, until I began my investigation – think they know about HRT is wrong on two counts: every form of HRT is not the same, and the terrifying cancer-scare headlines which erupted with the Women's Health Initiative Study back in 2002 refer to the older, synthetic forms of HRT that have now been superseded by a completely different products. It's not like comparing apples with pears; it's like comparing apples with plastic apples. The huge uptake around the world of plant-based, body-identical HRT (which from this point on I'll refer to as just body-identical HRT) is the beginning of a medical revolution that will have massive benefits in protecting women's long-term health.

Frustratingly, there is a cultural and medical resistance blocking natural hormone replacement: British and American doctors rely on outdated research on outdated forms of HRT, which was linked to a small increase in breast cancer. Breast cancer also has a totemic fear for women, striking at the very essence of femininity. One particular piece of research has generated more headlines than any other on the subject of HRT and breast cancer, and it's worth taking apart.

The Women's Health Initiative Scandal

On July 10, 2002, there were 13 million women happily on hormone replacement therapy in America[10] two million in the UK,[11] plus more all around the world. That morning, they woke up to a splash of terrifying front-page headlines: 'HRT study cancelled over cancer and stroke fears,' announced the *Guardian*; 'Alarm over HRT cancer risk,' reported the *Sydney Morning Herald*; 'HRT linked to breast cancer,' said the *Daily Mail*. The *New York Times* summed it up: 'Hormone replacement study a shock to the medical system.'

The reports were not merely a shock to the medical system, with some doctors ceasing to prescribe hormones altogether; they also, understandably, caused horror and panic among patients themselves. Many threw away their pills the morning the story broke and got their hot flushes back the next night. One million women eventually gave up HRT in the UK as a result of the announcements.[12] This was the most significant news story yet on HRT,[13] and the fallout has continued to reverberate ever since. The American Women's Health Initiative (WHI) was the largest women's health prevention study ever undertaken, with government backing, and studied 16,600 women on HRT.[14] The hastily announced results changed the future health of millions – mostly for the worse. The WHI is considered the Bible, the behemoth of HRT research, and continues to influence decisions about whether to replace women's decreasing hormones almost two decades on. But was the study reliable?[15] And why is it still being constantly cited by the NHS and applied to today's very different versions of HRT?

The first astonishing fact about the WHI study is that most of the participants *were not recently menopausal.* The average patient was aged 63, and some were as old as 79, with estrogen receptors that had probably packed up for good and would not be revived by the old oral, synthetic forms of HRT used in the trial. In addition, the majority were overweight or obese, and therefore already more prone to breast cancer. In order that the participants would not immediately spot the placebo pills, the study tried not to include any who had menopausal symptoms, such as hot flushes,[16] yet evidence has shown HRT is best started in the 'critical window',[17] when periods end, around the age of 51, while estrogen receptors are still functioning. 'In the WHI study, older women were suddenly being given relative overdoses of hormone therapy; most of them were twelve years post-menopause,' explains consultant gynaecologist Nick Panay. He runs the West London Menopause and Premenstrual Syndrome Service at Queen Charlotte's &

Chelsea and Chelsea & Westminster hospitals, and is about to head the International Menopause Society. 'The other frustrating thing was, when data was released across all age groups, it turned out that the 50–59 age group were doing well on HRT and the risks were very much within the older group.' This was not made clear in the initial WHI press announcement.

The next revelation was that all the estrogen HRT in the study was extracted from horse urine, in a pill called Premarin (*pre*gnant *mar*e's ur*in*e). As you might have guessed, horse estrogen isn't identical to ours. The other pill used in the study was a combined HRT called Prempro, which contained the horse urine along with – and this is a crucial point – a synthetic progestin called medroxyprogesterone acetate, which later turned out to be the suspected culprit in increased breast cancer cases.[18 19] Prempro caused a 29 per cent increase in heart attacks, a 41 per cent increase in strokes, and a 26 per cent increase in breast cancer, compared with the control group of participants.[20] Surprisingly, this pill is still being sold internationally. A new, low-dose version, Premique, with the same ingredients, is listed as one of the approved HRTs on the British National Formulary, the principal prescribing guide for medications available on the NHS.

As new studies emerged, and doubt was cast on the methodology and pharmacology of the WHI, there was increasing confidence in the new, body-identical forms of HRT. But the WHI study refused to go away and even appeared as part of a new report in *The Lancet* as recently as 2019, 'Type and Timing of Menopausal Hormone Therapy and Breast Cancer Risk'.[21] This was a number-crunching meta-analysis of previous investigations – including the original WHI study – by academics including Professor Valerie Beral, an epidemiologist at Oxford University, and also covered her own 'Million Women Study'.[22] They concluded that taking five years of HRT would increase breast cancer risk by 1 in 50 women taking the old combined estrogen and progestin pill. The news exploded again: 'Breast cancer risk from using HRT is "twice what was thought"' (*Guardian*), with the prize for the meanest headline going to the *Sunday Times*: 'Our obsession with youth brings too many HRT risks'.

But this time the response was very different from 2002. Now, a menopause movement existed, armed with medical expertise and reflected on social media. A bit like the 1998 anti-vax scandal that linked the MMR jab with autism in the same medical journal, the *Lancet* report met with rebuttals from doctors and academics because the work was based on old HRT and old studies that went as far back as 1981. Sadly, the NHS Medicines and Healthcare products Regulatory Agency sent out a panicked letter to doctors citing the 'new' *Lancet* research, and another clampdown on HRT prescriptions resulted. But it turned out that only 0.4 per cent of the women in Beral's meta-analysis[23] were using the safer, micronised progesterone and transdermal estrogen. Almost everyone was on the older forms of HRT.

Medical experts like the British Menopause Society agree that the newer, body-identical HRT is far more beneficial,[24] but the news doesn't seem to have dripped through the layers of NHS bureaucracy. In a 2020 joint statement,[25] the British, European, Australasian and International menopause societies and the Royal College of Obstetricians and Gynaecologists said: 'We believe that no arbitrary limits should be placed on the dose or duration of usage of menopausal hormone therapy.' But convincing ordinary women and GPs of the safety of newer forms of HRT is a thankless task, and it's a worldwide crisis, according to Professor Susan Davis, former president of the International Menopause Society in Australia. 'The trauma of the WHI study persists. A lot of that data is just appalling,' says Davis, damningly. 'There is still a huge push back against HRT: women think it's wrong, not for them, and they shouldn't have it unless they are desperate.' She sighs. 'It's like turning the *Titanic* – and pushing it uphill.'

What's in my HRT? Synthetic progestins v body-identical progesterone

Women need progesterone in HRT to protect their womb, as unopposed estrogen thickens the lining, risking uterine cancer.[26] But we're not in chemistry class here, so why should you care about the difference between synthetic progestins and natural, body-identical progesterone? In fact, that difference is crucial to women's health and the safer use of hormone replacement in the future. As any kid in first-year chemistry could tell you by looking at the diagram, body-identical progesterone is, as the name suggests, chemically and structurally the same as the hormone produced by your own body. Progestins, on the other hand, have a different structure, and may react differently with the body's progesterone receptors. It turns out that it is worth reading the ingredients on the packet, because the majority of HRT pills contain progestins – like the medroxyprogesterone acetate used in the WHI study, or norethisterone, levonorgestrel and desogestrel – and these showed a slightly increased risk of breast cancer[27] in an analysis of studies covering over 86,000 women, while HRT containing body-identical progesterone did not. 'The more you look at the WHI study, the more you see it is flawed,' says Professor Tony Howell, Chair in Breast Oncology at Manchester University and Professor of Medical Oncology at the city's Christie Hospital. 'The results refer to combined HRT with a nasty progestin, which is quite different from progesterone.'

Professor Howell instead recommends women take body-identical micronised progesterone alongside estrogen. 'The whole of HRT data suggests that progesterone is not causing breast cancer. The data on progesterone is reasonable. The "E3N" study in France showed progesterones were good, with no risk of breast cancer for five years, and that synthetic progestins were the nasty stuff, with a higher rate of cancer.[28] It's a good study. We should just get the good HRT stuff out there.' Quite simply, we should avoid synthetic progestins if possible (which are still in high doses in the contraceptive pill, but that's a whole other story) and stick to natural progesterone or dydrogesterone,[29] the one progestin that also has a safer profile.[30] A Mirena coil only contains tiny amounts of progestins, so is even safer than oral HRT.[31]

These are the British Menopause Society recommendations, co-authored by Nick Panay, consultant at the West London Menopause and Premenstrual Service: 'HRT regimens that included estrogen and micronised progesterone or dydrogesterone were not associated with an increased risk of invasive breast cancer with short-term use up to five years. Long-term use (more than five years) was associated with a small increase in the risk of breast cancer, but this risk was no longer statistically significant following discontinuation of HRT.'[32] This was based largely on the large 'E3N' study of the long-term health of around 80,000 French teachers who were either on HRT or nothing at all, where the risks of the different kinds of hormones used could be compared.[33] Some research is even more encouraging: a smaller study of 1,555 women, also in France, where micronised progesterone has been popular for years, showed that the use of this form of HRT actually *lowered* the risk of breast cancer by 20 per cent over four years, while the use of synthetic progestins increased the risk.[34] Another study, of 4,949 women, also showed no risk after two years with micronised progesterone.[35] The *Lancet* 'Type and Timing' report mentioned earlier found that the relative breast cancer risk for progesterone users was 9 per cent lower than for never-users of HRT.[36]

These studies confirm that progesterone is much safer and behaves very differently in the body from synthetic progestins.[37] Professor Frank Stanczyk of the Keck School of Medicine at University of Southern California and colleagues wrote a fascinating paper on this, proposing a theory why progestins are the problem ingredient in HRT: 'We hypothesize that estrogen acts via a mechanism that primes the tissue, and when progestins are added, there is a promotional effect resulting in increased breast cancer diagnosis.'[38] Another study swapped progestin-based HRT for a progesterone-based alternative, and women experienced fewer hot flushes, better sleep, and less anxiety and depression, with around 80 per cent saying they felt happier with progesterone.[39]

Some women have a progestin or progesterone intolerance

and find they cause depression, bloating and breast tenderness, which means it's hard to use HRT, but sometimes a Mirena coil can help, as can using progesterone in a lower dose, via vaginal pessaries. (I'd just like to put in a note for vegans here: while progesterone is plant-based, the coating on the widely used Utrogestan oral pill contains gelatin; however, there are other progesterone pessaries available without gelatin.)

So, there we are: the latest research shows that micronised progesterone is safer and easier to tolerate, and it can be used both orally and vaginally. In the UK, the main progesterone used is Utrogestan, while in the USA Prometrium is most widely given. Given the much safer profile of progesterone, you might think the NHS would be rushing to prescribe it, but – and this makes me want to scream with frustration – getting hold of Utrogestan turns out to be a nightmare postcode lottery for patients. There's a huge area of Britain in which Utrogestan isn't on the NHS-approved pharmaceutical formulary list as a menopause treatment, including parts of Scotland and many regions in the north, while it's much more easily available in, say, London. A campaign has started in Scotland to change this. The pharmaceutical company Theramex which makes HRT says that 10 per cent more of the older combined estrogen and progestin oral HRT is prescribed in the north of England, although a few savvy doctors in the 'banned' areas prescribe the better stuff 'off Formulary' – on the quiet. It is, indeed, grim Up North, and it's yet another injustice tossed on the pile.

The drug of choice in the private sector is body-identical HRT, so why are the majority of NHS prescriptions still for oral combined HRT with progestins? Panay explains:

'The older HRT formulations are relatively cheap and the big pharmaceutical companies will keep pumping them out until doctors and women ask for something better.' Indeed, oral combined HRT costs the NHS about £30 per year, while transdermal estrogen and separate micronised progesterone costs around £100.[40] Go figure.

Body-identical transdermal estrogen

Using body-identical transdermal estrogen after the age of 50 halves your chances of breaking a hip[41] and reduces your chances of having a heart attack.[42 43] I talked about the protective superpowers of transdermal estrogen in Chapter 3, but taking it also feels fantastic – a return to sanity – as menopausal symptoms disappear and your energy and strength returns. I have personally discovered that when HRT is good, it is very, very good. Like childbirth or an orgasm, you can't imagine it until you've tried it.

Body-identical transdermal estrogen comes as a patch, spray or rub-on gel applied to the skin. Some women love patches, although a few find they crumple, peel off or cause an allergic skin reaction. Davina McCall has done an entertaining YouTube video of her morning routine, where she demonstrates putting a see-through estrogen patch on her hip next to her tattoo.[44] I started with two pumps of estrogen gel a day, and now my GP has prescribed three pumps – or else my hot flushes threaten to reappear. The ability to easily vary the amount according to symptoms is particularly good for women during the fluctuations from the perimenopause to the menopause. Many women swapped to the gel after shortages in 2020 of HRT patches and other preparations, which the government did nothing about.[45] Women went to their pharmacist to get a prescription they had been on for years, and suddenly found it was unavailable. Patients were offered patches with lower or higher doses than they were used to, or oral HRT instead of transdermal, or nothing at all. 'The psychological impact of not being able to access hormone replacement has been devastating,' says menopause counsellor and #MakeMenopauseMatter campaigner Diane Danzebrink, whose Facebook The Menopause Support Network was filled for months with messages from panicking women.

The situation was so dire that the British Menopause Society, the Royal College of Obstetricians and Gynaecologists and its Faculty of Sexual and Reproductive Healthcare (FSRH) demanded an investigation from then secretary of state for health, Matt Hancock. Dr Asha Kasliwal, President of the FSRH, said: 'These shortages disproportionately affect the most vulnerable in our society, for example a woman struggling to access clinics, or a transgender patient, who is already under psychological distress, and for whom changing contraceptive preparations could cause further difficulties.'[46] For trans women taking HRT after surgery, that meant transition could suddenly stall.

The shortages were attributed to a problem with the glue that sticks the patches to the skin, but it turned out that the main roadblock was the NHS had changed its drug tariff, putting HRT in a new, cheaper category to manage costs. Manufacturers were unwilling to sell HRT in the UK at such low prices when markets in Europe and elsewhere were paying more. A combination of the new fixed-pricing system and the falling value of the pound meant that the UK was a less valuable market for manufacturers to allocate stock, leading to shortages. Would that happen to hormones like insulin for diabetics? Why is HRT considered to be about lifestyle rather than health? 'For many, it's led to a return of physical, psychological and cognitive symptoms,' says Danzebrink. 'Some women have resorted to buying their HRT products via private pharmacies, with some spending several hundred pounds since the shortages began. Others have travelled abroad or asked friends or family travelling or living abroad to buy HRT products over the counter for them.' Why is using HRT always such a struggle when it should be so simple?

The shortages came back with a vengeance in 2022, as more women turned to safer transdermal HRT, and even a temporary HRT 'Tsar' seemed unable to solve them. While some oral and equine estrogens like Prempro were shown to increase the risk of cardiovascular disease in women in the WHI study,[47] transdermal estrogen has a protective effect,[48] increasing good cholesterol, decreasing bad, and relaxing the blood vessels to help blood flow. Transdermal estrogen also prevents osteoporosis caused when hormones fail during the menopause. The average improvement in bone density is around 3.4 per cent after one year of transdermal estrogen, and 3.7 per cent after two years.[49] That's a miracle repair and renewal job; a complete reversal of fortune. As osteoporosis expert Professor David Reid told me: 'In women under sixty, particularly those with menopausal symptoms, transdermal HRT is a good option and they usually gain a bit of extra bone density.' Reid particularly recommends hormone replacement for the 1 per cent of patients with premature ovarian insufficiency (POI) under 40. Without treatment, women with early menopause will quickly have the crumbling bones of someone 10 or 20 years older.

For those on bone-sucking steroids, additional estrogen is essential. My friend Deb is in her fifties and on steroids for her back, but her GP (old, male) told her it was time to stop her HRT and refused to give her a new prescription until she got a second opinion. 'Is he quite mad?' I said, emailing her the official guidelines from the National Institute for Health and Care Excellence (NICE) to give him, which say: 'Explain to women that their risk of fragility fracture is decreased while taking HRT and that this benefit is maintained during treatment and may continue for longer in women who take HRT for longer.' 'FFS,' Deb wrote back.

The same head-in-the-sand view of transdermal estrogen goes right to the top. I was at a grand charity dinner for the Royal Osteoporosis Society in 2019, and there was the patron, HRH Camilla, Duchess of Cornwall, up on the big screen talking about her family's struggle with brittle bones. 'Sadly, as I grew older, I learned a great deal more about osteoporosis at first hand, as I watched both my mother and grandmother suffer the pain and ignominy of this agonising disease,' she said, detailing the horrifying experience of watching how her mother 'shrank' as she approached her last birthday, at 72, and encouraging donations for new research. Not a word was said by anyone about HRT – apart from at my table, which was full of menopause doctors and consultants tearing their hair out in frustration.

Encouragingly, in 2021 the Royal Osteoporosis Society (ROS) updated outdated advice on its website about HRT, and now explains that some types, particularly estrogen only, do not have a risk of breast cancer or blood clots. 'There have been many reports in the media about HRT and these have not always been accurate or balanced, causing worry and confusion about long term health risks. HRT is a safe and effective treatment [for osteoporosis] when it's prescribed in the right way for the women who need it.'[50]

Professor Reid said there needs to be more research. 'I would love to see a study comparing HRT and bisphosphonates in menopausal women, but it would probably cost £2 million over the years, and no one is going to fund that,' he said. Certainly not the drugs companies getting £9,000 a year for each woman on osteoporosis drugs, as opposed to the cost of just over £100 a year for HRT. Perhaps the Duchess of Cornwall can intervene? Can we write a new HRT scene into *The Crown*?

Testosterone

Treatment with testosterone is growing exponentially in private medicine and at a few specialist clinics providing NHS menopause care, and it's a secret every woman should know. At the menopause, testosterone replacement usually aims to achieve the level of a typical 40-something woman; younger women have twice that amount of testosterone. So, testosterone replacement does not suddenly cause male-pattern baldness, a hairy chest or a deep voice (unless you intentionally overdose). Better still, it's safe: testosterone does *not* increase the risk of breast cancer;[51] in fact, one small study showed that testosterone implants in menopausal women *reduced* the rate of breast cancer[52] – however, it is usually taken via a cream or gel through the skin (oral testosterone is not used as it can have an adverse effect on the liver). Doctors advise rubbing the cream on your inner thigh or abdomen, although I've met a couple of women who found that when they rubbed the gel on the same place on their leg every day, a patch of hair there became more luxuriant. Top tip: regularly move the application point around the body, perhaps to a visibly hairless area. But, sensibly used, it's not a problem: 'Supplementing testosterone at menopause won't make you grow a moustache,' reassures Nick Panay of the British Menopause Society.

Like a growing number of women, I use body-identical testosterone every day, not just for libido (although that's a delightful extra), but for the hormone's effects on cognition, muscle, mood, bone density and energy. I rub a pea-sized blob of AndroFeme testosterone cream (currently the only female testosterone cream available) onto my thigh, and I feel quite simply 'on it', as capable of creating and multitasking as I used to be. I doubt the battle to get this book on the shelves would have happened without that energy; the same goes for getting the accompanying menopause documentary off the ground during the Covid-19 pandemic – persuading TV companies to back a prime-time programme with the 'off-putting' word 'menopause' in the title was like nailing jelly to the wall, but we did it. When the menopause left me flat, testosterone helped me stand up again. In the words of Davina McCall, 53, our barnstorming presenter on the documentary: 'After I started taking testosterone, I walked into a television meeting and I felt empowered. I felt like I was thirty again.'

The advantage of a cream or gel is you can lower the dose

if you feel you need slightly less (and we should also acknowledge the dangers of taking too much). My friend Bindi, who was in an executive job with a bullying, tantrum-throwing boss before she went freelance, says: 'I didn't need the testosterone my doctor gave me very much – except on Sunday nights, before the brutal Monday-morning meeting.' Is the midlife testosterone fall-off one of the reasons there are still so few senior women on company boards? Is the glass ceiling hormonal as well as cultural? Are the successful women the ones whose testosterone remains naturally high?

Although it's hard for women to get testosterone on the NHS, it's not impossible if you have a sympathetic and well-informed GP, although there's ingrained resistance. In one survey, 68 per cent of UK health professionals said they wouldn't prescribe it to women.[53] That's despite the NICE guidelines for doctors that say, under 'Altered Sexual Function': 'Consider testosterone supplementation for menopausal women with low sexual desire if HRT alone is not effective.'[54] ('Consider' does not mean 'offer', so many women are refused. Plus there's no mention of testosterone's cognitive benefits.) Yet testosterone for women is only available 'off licence', since the hormone is licensed on the NHS only for men.

Dr Zoe Hodson, a former GP and now a menopause specialist in Manchester, has been campaigning to get testosterone for women on NHS formularies (the list of drugs doctors are advised to use) throughout the UK, and Carolyn Harris MP is also fighting for this in Parliament. Dr Hodson describes the barrier to the change: 'Consider that in ten years of my training and fifteen years of practice, not once was testosterone mentioned as a female hormone. There is absolutely *no* support for GPs to manage this, and they constantly face headlines telling them how dreadful doctors are. Why would they prescribe it?'

I made three attempts to get testosterone from my NHS practice. The first time, they suggested I take a particular old-style combined synthetic pill that has testosterone-like effects (despite not containing testosterone) but this pill carries an increased risk of stroke and breast cancer[55] compared with my own body-identical HRT. I turned the proffered pill down. On my second testosterone tackle, a few months later, my GP said she would have to refer the request up to a hospital ob-gyn. There was no reply, but a year later I asked for a referral to the NHS menopause clinic and got testosterone at last. I must add that my GP ought to know that testosterone is both safe and effective, since she is the designated 'menopause expert' at our big north-London practice. Added to which, why am I left feeling embarrassed about asking for testosterone, somehow unentitled, despite the hormone's clear mental and physical health benefits for me and most women in the short and long term? But it's not really doctors' fault, as the menopause medical education available is both limited and out of date. So I still pay for my testosterone cream privately and get the rest of my HRT on the NHS. But not everyone can. I use the Australian AndroFeme testosterone cream, which is made specially for women, and it costs me about £160 for a year's supply (some women need twice that amount). I'd rather spend money on that than a weekly latte from Starbucks, but we should be allowed our own hormone back, free of charge, like men are. Even if you do manage to get it on the NHS, it's still tricky, says Davina McCall, as the only available UK products are aimed at men: 'I have to work out what's a fifth of a man-sized pump of Testogel every day.'

Dr Hodson was working as a GP in Manchester when a worker from the local Tesco supermarket, in her late fifties, came in complaining of low libido. She was also forgetting everything and making mistakes at the till. She was already on estrogen and progesterone HRT, so Dr Hodson prescribed some testosterone gel to try 'off licence' on the NHS, since it was not on the approved drugs list for their area. 'Around fifteen per cent of prescriptions are "off licence", so this isn't exceptional, and I adhered to the British Menopause Society guidelines.' At this point, she had completed additional training in the menopause. 'I had always viewed testosterone as something that was complicated and had to be prescribed in a specialist clinic. It isn't.'

A few weeks later, news of the miracle improvement for the first woman had got around the whole supermarket, and another Tesco worker arrived at her surgery, then another. Three of them went on testosterone and Tesco's productivity probably took a leap upwards. But that wasn't all. Dr Hodson rang one of the women to enquire how she was getting on with the testosterone, and recalls, 'I just got a wicked giggle down the phone. Another woman told me: "I don't want to go back into the crazy-lady cupboard."' The Tesco checkout was not giving up its testosterone. On her @manchestermenopausehive Instagram, Dr Hodson posted a hippie-pink flower bearing the words 'Testosterone – It's Not Just For Boys'. She has run a campaign with Menopause Support[56] to get women who are refused testosterone to write to their local clinical commissioning group asking for the hormone to be put on the approved drugs list for their area, citing the science behind their request. 'I firmly believe that testosterone should not just be available to the affluent or ultra-persistent, and I'm determined to end health inequalities in this area,' says Dr Hodson. 'Why do women have to grovel to retrieve their brains, energy and a semblance of sex drive in 2021?'

It turns out there was, for a while, a testosterone patch in circulation in the UK and Europe called Intrinsa, licensed as safe for women by the European Medicines Agency in 2006, but which was withdrawn by the manufacturers in 2012 'because the product was not commercially viable',[57] i.e. not enough patches were being prescribed by doctors. The Food and Drug Administration in America turned down Intrinsa in the shadow of the WHI, yet the makers Procter & Gamble had data from two large trials demonstrating the safety and efficacy of their product. In one 24-week study of 533 women, those taking Intrinsa reported a 51 per cent increase in frequency of 'satisfying sexual activity' and a 49 per cent improvement in sexual desire, compared with their previous experience.[58]

In terms of sexual desire, testosterone is of huge importance for younger women who have an early or medically-induced menopause, and for a while the patch was offered for that. Dr Rebecca Gibbs is an ob-gyn consultant at the Royal Free Hospital in London and a volunteer for The Daisy Network, which supports women with premature ovarian insufficiency. 'I do live chats online to help members, and some aren't even offered testosterone and others are on a normal dose for fifty-year-old women, but they're twenty-five and suffering, with no libido and should have much more,' says Gibbs. 'I learned nothing about testosterone for women at medical school or postgrad, but I decided to do advanced training skills as a menopause specialist at the Whittington Hospital Menopause Clinic. The women who ask for testosterone have usually done their own research. The classic patient coming in is a woman at the peak of her career, promoted as high as she can go, managing a couple of teenagers, and just exhausted.'

The call for testosterone to be made freely available goes from the cutting edge of menopause research to the reassuringly normal world of daytime television. Lorraine Kelly, who presents *Lorraine* on ITV every weekday, first spoke on air about taking HRT herself in 2017, and said the discussion with the show's resident doctor 'got the biggest reaction we've had on anything. It touched a nerve. We need to keep it in the public eye and get women angry. I'm banging the drum for this.' She uses testosterone herself and said: 'The unfairness is that most women can't get it at all. We're right at the bottom of the bloody list.'

The difficulty of getting (good) HRT

So why is it so difficult to get HRT in the UK, particularly the best kind? The 'gold standard' prescribed by NHS and private menopause experts is plant-based, body-identical transdermal estrogen in gel, patches or spray, coupled with body-identical progesterone in a pill, vaginal pessary – or a Mirena coil. Add testosterone gel or cream to that, and you have the safest package.[59] As I've mentioned before, it is better if possible to avoid oral combined HRT containing synthetic progestins and estrogen which have a very small but increased risk of breast cancer, blood clots and stroke.

I use the 'gold standard', body-identical HRT myself, so let me take you on the journey that got me where I am today – healthy, happy and relatively sane. At 51, as I became increasingly boiling and bonkers but still had occasional periods, I went to the GP's surgery and was sent to the practice nurse, who gave me a Mirena coil, which releases small amounts of progestin directly into your womb, also acting as a form of contraception. I tried that, to no avail. The amounts of hormones in it are minuscule. Of course, I now know my body was also screaming for estrogen, but that wasn't on offer; the idea of full-blown HRT as I was only just starting the menopause was briskly brushed away by the nurse. Besides, I thought back then that HRT was the risky, weird option, and that I was the sort of person who would cope without drugs. I went the alternative route and splashed out in Holland & Barrett on St John's wort and a smorgasbord of herbal menopause supplements. I also ate soy beans and miso soup for months, hoping the phytoestrogens in them would percolate my body. Nothing helped. My periods stopped. I struggled on, until vanity intervened: my hair started to fall out in the shower.

This was a different level of emergency. I called my friend Deb. She said: 'You need this special HRT. I'm on it. We're all on it. Nobody talks about it.' I went to the London private clinic she suggested. I know that most people don't have the £300 that the initial consultation cost me – which is why I'm now campaigning for better access to HRT on the NHS. And I have since discovered the very serious risks (more of which later) of unlicensed private prescriptions. I was prescribed a combination of estrogen, testosterone and progesterone, and suddenly my life came back into focus. The hot flushes ended, my joints stopped hurting, my adrenaline-pumping anxiety disappeared and my heart stopped its erratic palpitations. And – I knew you'd want to know – my hair got thick again, while the wine-dark shadows beneath my eyes disappeared. I slept and slept and slept. I felt so much happier, and at last I had the energy to sort out the chaos of my life.

From a place of relative sanity and calm, I looked back on what had happened and was astonished that in both my visits to the GP's surgery – first for heart palpitations, and then for hot flushes and anxiety – HRT was not offered as an option, when it was so instantly effective. What happened to all the other women who were turned away and didn't have the money to join the privileged club of private HRT users? Later, when I found out about the safest body-identical HRT, I realised I could get it from my NHS doctor, and wondered why it was not being prescribed everywhere.

Despite the many and significant benefits of body-identical HRT, it remains out of reach to the majority of the population – and this is causing a national health crisis. I talk regularly to menopause specialists in the NHS and in private care, and every day they find themselves mopping up the mess after women are refused HRT in an initial consultation. Of course, some GPs and nurse practitioners are brilliant and well-informed, and many trainees are keen to learn, but there's a generation of doctors, gynaecologists and endocrinologists who have always worked in the shadow of the 2002 WHI report, which said that HRT increased the risk of breast cancer, and so are very reluctant to prescribe it.

Mandy Walker, 52, a care manager in Shropshire, went to

her GP when struggling with perimenopausal symptoms and was told: 'You can't have HRT because you'll get breast cancer and I'll be sued.' She tried another GP, who said: 'Go home, have a glass of wine, read a book, and be glad you're alive.'

One GP and menopause specialist shared with me a litany of her recent cases (anonymous), all of whom had been denied help before coming to her private clinic. Here are five examples:

'Woman with surgical menopause and raised body mass index was told by the gynaecologist who did her surgery that she didn't need estrogen replacement as she had enough fat of her own to provide her with it.'

'Woman in her early sixties who had requested and been denied HRT for twelve years, for symptoms and to prevent osteoporosis (as her mum had osteoporosis), diagnosed with osteoporosis and then still denied, so had to come to us to get HRT.'

'Woman in her mid-fifties with ten-year history of significant mental health issues. On multiple medication; stopped working and marriage broke up. She got substantially better with HRT very quickly. She feels very aggrieved for all she lost, and that nobody had ever considered her hormones.'

'Woman aged twenty-three with premature ovarian insufficiency told by endocrinologist that her early menopause and resulting fertility issues were irrelevant as she is in a same-sex relationship. Despite multiple requests to her GP and a further referral to NHS, still refused adequate treatment as needs a higher dose of HRT due to her age.'

And the most shocking:

'Woman who was told by the surgeon who removed her

ovaries that she didn't need hormones and just to think of it like a Labrador being spayed.'

I felt sick after hearing that, and fortunately that last particular patient managed to get HRT privately. However, few can do that. A survey published in 2020 by the British Journal of Medical Practice showed women were 29 per cent less likely to get HRT on the NHS in socio-economically deprived areas, and even if they did get help, their doctors tended to prescribe the cheaper, oral estrogen, which can cause blood clots, rather than the safer transdermal version.[60] As Dr Sarah Hillman, a co-author of the survey report, confirms: 'Women in deprived areas are more likely to suffer from strokes, diabetes and cardio-vascular problems, yet they are least likely to get transdermal HRT which would help.'

Dr Gibbs is of British Caribbean origin and works on the NHS's Workforce Race Equality Standard. She recalls: 'When I worked at the NHS menopause clinic in the Whittington Hospital, it was mostly a self-selecting group of middle-class white women who came in, who had already negotiated with their GPs to get there. The white wealthy either know exactly what they want or have gone privately first, had positive results and want the same on the NHS. The local Black and Asian community just don't seem to be coming in there.

'I also worked at the Royal London Hospital in London with a big Bangladeshi community, and women would come in talking of "all-over body pain, my teeth hurt, my head hurts, my hair hurts". Those are all menopausal symptoms, plus depression, and no one is giving them HRT. Black and Asian women are harder hit by osteoporosis, strokes and dementia, the risks of which can all be mitigated by HRT. It's economic sense, therefore, to see that prescribing HRT in the first place would save the NHS a lot in the future.'

There is a massive chasm between the have-HRTs and the have-nots, in terms of class and ethnicity. Let's take a peek for a moment into the hormone hall of fame: fans of HRT include Angelina Jolie, Oprah Winfrey, Kim Cattrall, Margaret Thatcher, Mariella Frostrup, Edwina Currie, Zoe Ball, Dawn French, Jenny Eclair, Bobbi Brown, Gabby Logan, Jane Seymour, Lorraine Kelly and Meg Mathews, all of whom have been positive and upfront about speaking out about HRT. But there many women in the public eye who keep their HRT habit hidden, and more openness would make a big difference. You can see at a glance which women are taking hormones: the runners, the city executives, the actresses, many of whom have private specialists. HRT flows in the very bloodstream of Hollywood, the Square Mile and Wall Street, but no one talks about it publicly. As Dr Louise Newson wryly notes: 'I can spot whether a woman is on HRT the minute she walks into the room, and it is not just about appearance but confidence.'

Hormone replacement therapy is a chaotic lottery, in which only those who can afford private medicine consistently win. If most women find it a struggle to get help, how hard must it be for those who are differently abled, in prisons, or otherwise excluded? In an article in the British Menopause Society journal,[61] David Martin discussed how menopause affects women with learning disabilities and laments that it is a neglected area of research: 'Menopause is usually earlier in women with learning disabilities and earlier still for those with Down's syndrome, but difficulties in understanding and communication mean that additional supports are often required. Debate about HRT often ignores the needs of women with learning disabilities who, as a result, are very often excluded from the decision-making process.' There is now a resource pack available for carers supporting women with learning disabilities through menopause.[62]

For most women, starting HRT isn't simple and often requires more than one visit to the GP. Dr Zoe Hodson explains 'You don't just prescribe HRT and leave women to it. They may need their progesterone or estrogen raised or lowered, to get it just right for them.' Women in their forties usually start on cyclical HRT, taking estrogen every day, and progesterone for the last 14 days of their cycle, with means they continue to have regular periods. Later, when periods stop, women usually change to continuous HRT, which provides a steady flow of hormones. As we know from the many forms of the contraceptive pill, women have very different reactions to the same hormones, and many women starting HRT find at first experience unexplained bleeding, period-like pains or enlarged breasts. 'Usually those symptoms settle down, but we need to be vigilant,' says Hodson. 'It takes time, and I often find there's trauma coming up in midlife that women are dealing with, and HRT is not an overnight cure.'

So, we need a professional follow-up, which many GPs are not yet equipped to give, so they will often refer women to a specialist menopause clinic. In 2021, there were 95 NHS menopause clinics in the UK, and yet there are 13 million women of menopausal age and older. The waiting times are often enormous. For my fellow journalist Amanda, who refused to go private, it took over a year to get an NHS appointment at a London menopause clinic. (And after eventually finding an estrogen patch that worked for her, she was hit by HRT shortages a few months later.) I asked followers on my @menoscandal Instagram how long they had waited for an HRT consulation at an NHS menopause clinic, and answers flooded in from around the country: eighteen months in Maidstone in Kent, a year in Stoke-on-Trent, nine months in Leicester, seven months in Edinburgh, three months in Newcastle, and one that just sadly said: 'Don't even have a clinic here in North Wales. GP just doesn't want to know.'

The toll of ignoring body-identical HRT

During my research, I came across a brilliant infographic created by Women's Health Concern and the British Menopause Society titled 'Understanding the Risks of Breast Cancer',[63] which is worth looking up. Based on the 2015 NICE guidelines, it explains the chances of people, like me, aged 50–59, developing breast cancer in the next five years, with little images of women lined up in a row. Obviously, cancer is an unpredictable act of God or genes, but lifestyle factors are incredibly important too.

The bad news:

- In the general population, 23 cases of breast cancer will be diagnosed per 1,000 women.
- If women take the old, synthetic HRT, an additional 4 cases appear.
- If women drink a large glass of wine every day, an additional 5 cases appear.
- If women are obese (BMI over 30), an additional 24 cases appear.

The good news:

- If women take 2.5 hours of moderate exercise per week, 7 cases disappear.
- If women take estrogen-only HRT, 4 cases disappear.

There's no information in the diagram on what happens if you take the new, body-identical HRT but a major French study showed no breast cancer risk over five years, and a tiny one over ten.[64] In 2022, research on almost half a million women and their prescriptions in the UK Clinical Research Practice Datalink[65] showed that estrogens were not associated with an increased risk of breast cancer, and micronised progesterone actually lowered the risk a tiny amount. The authors concluded that micronised progesterone was safer than synthetic progestins. And for women who no longer have a womb, estrogen-only HRT has been proven to reduce the chances of breast cancer in some studies,[67] while others show that women who use HRT will live four years longer than those without.[69]

Let's apply the above information to me. It would appear that I have no, or maybe a one in 1,000, extra risk of breast cancer because I have been taking body-identical HRT[70] for over five years. But because I exercise every day, I'm lowering my chances by seven, and because I don't drink, I'm lowering my risk even further. My reasons to take HRT are powerful: I also have Alzheimer's in my family – on top of which, all women have a one in five chance of developing the disease – and estrogen has a protective effect against it. HRT also helps prevent osteoporosis, which brings a one in two chance of breaking a bone, and lowering the chances of those two diseases is another huge positive for me. So there you have it – that's my rationale for staying on

HRT for the rest of my life. Aside from HRT keeping me sane and free of menopausal symptoms.

But the more time I spend in the gladiatorial menopause arena, the more I realise I'm one of the extremely lucky ones, who have found the right HRT and the access to it. Near where I grew up in Glasgow, the story is very different. Dr Helen Smith is a GP in her fifties working in Kilmarnock, where there are significant pockets of deprivation and a serious drugs problem, and 25 per cent of children are below the poverty line. Dr Smith trained in the era of the WHI study and says, 'It's been a very difficult thing to shake off, and it continues today as doctors my age are training the GPs of the future.' She says it is difficult to assess menopause needs in a ten-minute consultation, though consulting during the Covid-19 pandemic remotely, by Zoom or phone, gave her more of an opportunity to chat for longer. But the economic inequality in her community remains: 'A lot of middle-class people will go away and do their own research . . . and go in and ask for what they want, and the rich people will go private. So many of my patients have lots of difficulties in their lives already. They come from a very different place, with significant adverse childhood experiences, domestic abuse, alcohol and significant drug issues. If they can't afford data on their phones to educate their children, they won't be downloading a menopause app, will they?'

Dr Smith thinks menopause knowledge should begin in primary school sex education classes, in workplaces and in the doctor's surgery, with a simple list of symptoms for women. There's a double stigma for her patients around HRT – the suspicions about breast-cancer risk and the image problem – the fact that, as Dr Smith explains, 'it automatically puts you in the "older lady" zone. You also don't see any working-class women talking about menopause, so it's about role models.' (Actually, presenter Lorraine Kelly is a local example, having grown up in a 'single end', a one-room flat in Glasgow's Gorbals area.) Dr Smith also knows some older, male doctors who refuse to prescribe HRT altogether. The mental health burden in these deprived communities is higher too; Smith says that 'people will take antidepressants more often without question and often have been on them for other things earlier in life.'

Even when a woman asks for HRT, the struggle is not yet over for doctors in Scotland. The Greater Glasgow NHS drugs list of the prescriptions doctors should use first advises oral combined HRT tablets – a very bad idea for a deprived population already over-prone to clots, cancer and strokes, and most in need of the safest medicine. It doesn't quite fit with physicians' Hippocratic Oath: 'I will follow that system of regimen which, according to my ability and judgement, I consider for the benefit of my patients, and abstain from whatever is deleterious and mischievous.' Although her computer lights up with a red 'off licence' warning when she prescribes the safer HRT, Dr Smith says she goes ahead. 'If a woman needs it, then I'll do anything that minimises potential risk, and the risk depends on each individual.' A woman's life expectancy in the Kilmarnock area is 79 years old, compared with 85 in London.

There are many pioneers out there like Dr Smith, doing their best for women, in a secret revolution. 'There's a menopause movement among GPs who are educating themselves,' Smith says. 'There's an underworld. They are doing everything they can on the quiet for the menopause – but policy needs to catch up.'

If we apply the Hippocratic Oath to giving care to women

who have surgical or early menopauses, taking HRT is not a lifestyle choice; it is a matter of life and death. Professor Philip Sarrel of the departments of Obstetrics and Gynecology and Psychiatry at Yale University School of Medicine conducted a study in 2013 of how many American women died unnecessarily because they threw away their HRT after the shock headlines from the Women's Health Initiative in 2002. Back then, around 90 per cent of hysterectomised women took HRT and many of them must have been among the two million Americans who stopped taking hormones. (Statistics show that in 2001, almost 18 million Americans had a least one prescription of HRT, and by 2008 it was less than 6 million.[71]) Over the ten years after the WHI study, Professor Sarrel estimates, there were between 18,000 and 91,000 excess early deaths from cardiovascular and other diseases for women with hysterectomies in the 50–59 age group. The damage would have been prevented by HRT – and, indeed, their life expectancy would have improved.[72]

Professor Sarrel says that in the USA one third of women have a hysterectomy by the time they are 50, and nowadays most are left high and dry without hormones. 'The cost tolls to the health system are massive, and human toll is unimaginable.' Yet somehow, the happiness and health of ageing women does not seem to be a priority in the America or the UK, and the latest accurate scientific information appears not to have percolated the sluggardly bureaucracy of the NHS or insurance companies, most of whom do not cover menopause. Yet it could save them all billions in long-term health care.

I'm not in the pay of any pharmaceutical companies, but I have researched everything I can about the safer, body-identical

HRT, and that's why I am evangelical about its benefits. I've met the scientists and doctors, read the research papers, cited the footnotes, talked to the patients and even tried various forms of HRT myself, and what I've found is what all the experts from the International, British, Australasian and European menopause societies have been saying for years:[73] body-identical HRT is better news, and every woman should have access to it if she wants.

9

THE RISKY BUSINESS OF MENOPAUSE

When the medical establishment is so set in its ancient ways, women have to find alternative routes to get what they need. Sometimes that means sharing information on social media, and sometimes that means taking other paths to hormone replacement. Since the coronavirus pandemic, patients have used telemedicine more confidently with their GPs, and there are huge numbers of private menopause clinics now going online. But what's safe, and whom to trust? Hormones are not Lemsip and every woman is different. Some may have problems with absorbing estrogen, others with tolerating progesterone. Mismanagement of hormone treatment can have serious consequences.

While younger women have found better understanding and health activism through the period poverty and period power movements, coupled with useful menstrual health apps like Clue and Flo period trackers, femtech for the menopause – menotech – is just starting up. It's not yet clear what the market will look like, but billions are being invested in it. The already-established Balance Menopause Support app is free, medically accurate and has over 250,000 users internationally, and there are other UK-based advice sites like M-Powered and Gen-M. The UK-based Health & Her[1] website is filled with advice from nutritionists, relationship counsellors and even make-up artists, and sells dozens of menopausal herbal remedies, as well as doctors' video consultations at £95 for 30 minutes.

High-street chemist Superdrug offers 'Online Doctor' consultations where you can just fill in an email form, which is checked by a doctor, and get HRT sent to your door.[2] It's not cheap, though – progesterone pills and estrogen patches cost about five times the amount you would pay for an NHS prescription. I asked the Superdrug press office if there was a gap in the market, where women were not getting the service they needed from their own GPs. They replied: 'Yes, there were, and still are, access issues with women telling us they're unable to get through to their usual doctor for a prescription, but also with supply; we have had a lot of women unable to get their usual prescription [patches] and so they turned to us for this or an equivalent.' Superdrug said they provided information on the website 'which allows women to make an informed decision, but if they have questions, they can message our doctors non-urgently through their account, or arrange a £25 telephone consultation with one of us to discuss things further.' I asked if those doctors are menopause specialists. 'While not all of us are trained GPs, we are all trained in menopause and HRT prescribing, and so any one of us would be comfortable consulting with women about this issue.'

That is not entirely reassuring in terms of expertise, and doctors or prescribing nurses will not be able to pick up visual signals in a standard email – and women themselves may not tell the whole story. Even a Zoom consultation is better than this, and everyone's first resort for safety reasons should be their GP's surgery – that's assuming that the doctor will be willing to prescribe HRT.

The menopausal gold rush is about to begin, with Generation X being digitally literate and willing to try online clinics. In America, menopause telemedicine site Gennev[3] was set up by Microsoft executive Jill Angelo and former Neutrogena executive Jacqui Brandwynne with a mission to 'empower every woman to take control of her health in the second half of life'. It raised £2.9 million in investment seed-money and now provides online appointments with menopause-certified ob-gyns that can be paid through health insurance, plus coaching with registered dietitians, wellness products, community and free education. The US Peanut menopause app connects an online community. The American investment group Female Founders Fund[4] says that 'women's health has outgrown its perception as a "niche" area of healthcare and developed into a key area of interest for investors.' Over the past five years, over $1 billion has been invested in women's health companies in the US. Only 5 per cent of the femtech start-ups are for menopause, but that's growing. Female Founders estimates the menopause to be a $600 billion market in the future.

I can't help thinking that much of this is profiteering, and that if women were given proper choices and care on the NHS in the UK, and from health insurers in America, it would be unnecessary. We don't need more menopause products – sweat-wicking nighties, hot-flush-predictor wristbands or potions for symptoms. We just need to recognise that for most women menopause symptoms are an easily treated hormonal deficiency, and the transition is much easier once those problems are solved.

I know that now, of course, but a few years ago I was taken in by the soft sell of the menopause industrial complex myself. I turned to the private sector after logging into the NHS website in peak menopausal panic and searching 'HRT'. This is what came up: 'Find out about hormone replacement therapy (HRT) – how it can help menopausal symptoms, the different types of HRT, and what the main risks and side effects are – including how it can raise your risk of breast cancer.'[5]

I was petrified. I wasn't going to click any further into the website to find out precisely how HRT could raise my risk of breast cancer. And there was no information on the availability of NHS-regulated, body-identical HRT and its lower risks. I didn't know it existed. My bursting Pandora's box of menopausal symptoms led me to investigate privately available bioidentical compounded hormones – 'compounded' meaning they are titrated in quantities specific to each person (note, this isn't the same as the regulated body-identical hormones you get on the NHS). Like hundreds of thousands of women in the UK and over 18 million in America,[6] I thought compounded hormones would do the trick. Once they'd slunk out of the menopausal closet, three of my hardest-working friends swore by compounded hormones, describing them as life-changing and definitely worth the £300 initial private consultation fee. 'After all, some women pay £300 for lip filler,' said one journalist, who'd panicked after she thought she was losing her memory and her job, 'and this is salvation for the same amount.'

Bear with me, because I know private medicine is the route for the privileged, but it is also increasingly the last resort for women who have been wrongly refused HRT by their GPs or those on a long waiting list for NHS a menopause clinic. I've talked to women who have crowdfunded cash from girlfriends and relatives, and maxed-out credit cards, to get private help. Personally, I thought I was taking the sensible route, avoiding the vajazzled beauty clinics that offered 'anti-ageing hormones' as part of Botox, filler and labiaplasty packages. Instead I googled the more reputable-looking clinics in London, which are mostly staffed by qualified doctors and specialists. Their websites are well-designed, reassuring havens of calm. Take the London Hormone Clinic in Harley Street,[7] which says: 'As bioidentical hormones have the same chemical structure to our own hormones, they can act in our bodies like the real hormones we produce, unlike synthetic hormone like substances found in HRT and the pill.'

That's encouraging, I thought. Natural hormone replacement therapy sounds much less dangerous. I also looked at The Marion Gluck Clinic, in Wimpole Street, which pioneered bioidentical hormone replacement therapy (BHRT) in the UK. 'We take a personalised approach, providing bespoke medicine tailored to you and your needs,' the clinic says on its website, 'because there is no such thing as a "one-size fits all" approach to health. BHRT is very effective at enhancing quality of life, slowing down ageing and improving wellbeing.'[8] Bespoke! The Marion Gluck Clinic offers a 'female hormone profile' blood test to check your depleted levels and then tops them up with compounded hormones in the form of a cream or a lozenge that you slowly melt in your mouth, each tailored to each menopausal woman.

As I investigated further, I found an article in the *Guardian*[9] by Jeanette Winterson, an author I whose work I have read voraciously since her novel *Oranges Are Not the Only Fruit*. For Winterson, it turned out that Synthetic Was Not the Only HRT. Never base your medical decisions on literary taste, but I was fascinated by the *Guardian* piece in which Winterson interviewed the pioneering Dr Marion Gluck, who differentiated Big Pharma HRT from the natural stuff: '[Synthetic] HRT is ham-fisted,' said Gluck. 'It's like trying to perform surgery with a mallet. We don't need to flood our bodies with synthetic hormones.' Winterson's testimonial ended with her tanking up on the compounded hormones and saying: 'I feel at home in my body again.'

In the end, I went to a clinic recommended by friends, enjoyed the soothing mood-music in the elegant waiting room and partook of all the free healthy snacks and herbal teas to try to get my money's worth. I met the menopause doctor, who seemed very sensible and still worked part-time for the NHS. Unlike the short, ten-minute visits to my GP, she took time to ask in a holistic way about my health and habits, and she explained bioidentical compounded hormones very clearly. I had a blood test where we discovered my levels of estrogen, progesterone and testosterone were comically low, and I was prescribed a small pump of cream containing all three hormones, to rub on my wrist morning and night. I could hardly wait. After all, none other than Oprah Winfrey had declared, 'After one day on bioidentical estrogen, I felt the veil lift.'

Then came my own 'take up thy damp sheets and walk' miracle moment as the hormones irrigated the desert of my body and the hot flushes, night sweats, anxiety and heart palpitations disappeared. At the end of one week, I saw myself in the mirror and thought: you look healthy! By the end of the month, my joints had stopped hurting and my muscles had become elastic again. I ran a 10k race in Regent's Park, where I was given a medal and a banana for finishing.

I stayed on the cream for a year until my hormones really hit rock bottom. Then the clinic changed my prescription over to stronger lozenges that you cut into smaller squares and allowed to melt in your mouth twice a day. All was well, until I got a new batch of lozenges, labelled with the same prescription, posted out by the same private pharmacy that had been compounding (personalising) my dose. They tasted different. A few weeks after, I started to get irregular vaginal bleeding. I kind of ignored it, because women's lives are full of mysterious menstruation. Then I woke up one morning in a blood-boltered bed, and realised, *This isn't just a period that's turned up two years late.*

The hormone clinic seemed concerned – so concerned that they took my credit card details upfront and charged me around £600 for a blood test and a pelvic ultrasound, to examine what was going on in my uterus. The doctor checked to see if my womb lining might have thickened, which causes bleeding. She decided it was slightly thickened 'but within normal limits' and told me to stay on the lozenges. But she also charged me over £100 for a new prescription with a different mix. The bleeding went on, sporadically but lessened. The clinic said it would settle down.

It didn't. A month later, I went to my NHS GP in growing fear. She did a cervical smear and I handed over the compounded HRT lozenges, which I was still taking, and asked her what to do. She was in her twenties. She shrugged: 'I don't know much about that.' But my smear looked suspicious, and soon I was heading to my nearest hospital for a colposcopy – a microscopic examination of your cervix – and a hysteroscopy, where they stick a tiny camera up into your womb and look around.

'You're on the cancer test fast-track so you'll be seen within two weeks, but don't worry,' said my GP.

Fuck.

I ended up having two biopsies – to check for womb cancer and cervical cancer. I can't fault the NHS for kindness and efficiency, but when I showed the obstetrics and gynaecology consultants in the colposcopy and hysteroscopy departments my compounded HRT lozenges, printed with the exact quantities of the three hormones, both doctors just glanced at the packet and told me to keep on taking them if I felt okay.

The results of the biopsies were due in a few weeks. Here's a strange thing: as I waited, I wasn't as freaked out as I'd expected. It helped that I was with a new and supportive partner, who said encouragingly: 'Even if you were bald, I'd still love you,' although I reckoned it was more likely a hysterectomy was on the cards. A friend had suffered similar bleeding and had a hysterectomy just a month before. We'd just been for a slow walk-of-recovery on Wandsworth Common, and she was already back working part-time, but I saw how devastating the surgery could be. Still, I put the biopsies to the back of my mind and carried on.

The fact is, we're used to this. Women just live with ongoing biological catastrophes, from endometriosis to cystitis to postnatal depression. Although the term 'keeping mum' means keeping silent and actually refers to medieval mummers or players, the modern art of keeping mum is about denying your own gynaecology and not letting on to anyone about the chaos down below, particularly the shame of menopause. Things I've kept mum about – particularly at work – include: early miscarriage, abortion, tsunami periods, bleeding during pregnancy, postpartum stitch-ups, epic urinary tract infections, breast lump scares and, of course, postmenopausal bleeding. Most women have a similar list. It's all part of the rich, shitty tapestry of reproduction.

When I got the test results, I rejoiced. The biopsies weren't cancerous – although my cervix had a few dodgy-looking cells they would keep an eye on. But I was still worried about the compounded HRT, given that the consultants had not suggested I stopped. A few days later I saw my friend Kirsty Lang, who is a BBC radio presenter and always incredibly well-informed about everything. I told her what had happened. She said: 'Throw away that bioidentical compounded stuff immediately. It could have any old crap in it. It could have been compounded in an unlicensed pharmacy.'

Why hadn't the consultants known that, never mind my GP? Were the consultants in such separate silos they only looked for signs of cancer, and nothing beyond? Or did no one know what compounded HRT was? Did they think it was some kind of herbal remedy or sweeties? And what went on in some of these compounding pharmacies?

I immediately dumped the bioidenticals and went cold

turkey – actually roasting turkey – freaking out like an extra from *Trainspotting*. Kirsty – whose own story is in the coming chapter on the menopause and breast cancer – told me to get safer, NHS-approved hormones. She sent me off to Dr Louise Newson, who was then a stranger but who became an inspiration, a friend, and my go-to medical expert in all things menopause. There's nothing Louise likes better than emailing you an obscure scientific paper from the journal *Climacteric* at midnight. When I first met her in 2019, her practice had recently moved to Stratford-upon-Avon to become the Newson Health Menopause & Wellbeing Centre. The clinic is just along the road from Shakespeare's house, where Anne Hathaway must have braved her very own menopause around 1606, sweating it out in the second-best bed. (Where's the blue plaque for that, I ask you?)

At the clinic, Dr Newson turned out to be calm and reassuring, and appeared on the surface to be the sort of mum-of-three you might find glowing in the pages of a Waitrose magazine or the Boden catalogue. Once I got to know her, I noticed she often begins a sentence: 'I'm not really a feminist but . . .' In fact, she is a menopause revolutionary – media-savvy with a steel-trap scientific mind. I wasn't the first case of compounded hormone chaos Dr Newson had investigated, or the last. 'We see lots of women here who've spent huge amounts of money on these products and experienced numerous side effects.'

She explained that, quite simply, my progesterone and estrogen levels were out of sync, and I needed more progesterone to protect the lining of my womb and stop the bleeding. The hospital consultants should have known that. 'Bleeding often happens to women starting HRT and we can balance it out by changing the quantities,' Dr Newson told me. 'But with compounded hormones, you have no idea whether the amount you're getting is what it says on the packet, particularly if the pharmacy is unlicensed. You must have had too little progesterone and too much estrogen, even after they changed the dose. Every patient is different, and if the womb isn't properly protected by progesterone, that's a uterine cancer risk.' I've since met lots of other women in my research who have had similar 'cancer test fast-track' experiences to mine after starting HRT, and have just been on too little progesterone. It's great that the NHS takes the uterine cancer risk so seriously, but no one seems to be looking at the HRT element.

Taking compounded HRT isn't like just swallowing a pill. You are supposed to keep the lozenge in your cheek for about five or ten minutes, until it melts and goes into your bloodstream, but what if you accidentally swallow it before it's melted? To top it all, it turned out that compounded hormones are no more regulated than vitamins, despite being handed out by doctors in a white coat.

Dr Newson prescribed estrogen gel and micronised progesterone, explaining that they were licensed by the Medicines and Healthcare products Regulatory Agency and manufactured under strict regulation for use on the NHS, and that in future I could get them from my own GP. 'So none of this need have happened?' I asked her, gobsmacked. 'My GP could have given me this natural stuff, safely, three years ago, when I went in with the heart palpitations?' She answered, 'Yes, of course. But most GPs and ob-gyns get taught hardly anything about HRT prescription. There's no compulsory menopause module for GPs. I didn't get taught anything about menopause at medical school. I had to take a course myself, afterwards.' Dr Newson has now created her own 90-minute HRT prescribing webinar for doctors with FourteenFish medical education, which you can watch on YouTube.[10] With not-for-profit Newson Health Research and Education, she also developed the online professional Confidence in the Menopause Course, which is available for free on the FourteenFish website and now over 15,000 doctors and healthcare professionals have signed up.

After meeting Dr Newson I found a survey of doctors and nurses in the *British Journal of Family Medicine* from 2018 that showed 48 per cent had no training in managing the menopause, and 25 per cent said they were not confident prescribing HRT to menopausal women.[11] If doctors are lacking confidence, what hope is there for patients? It's even more shocking in America. A survey of junior doctors at 20 hospitals revealed that only 7 per cent thought they were 'adequately prepared to manage women in the menopause'.[12] Are the other 93 per cent just guessing? In any other area of medicine, this would be a scandal.

When Dr Newson realised that there was a huge gap in menopause care, she tried to set up an NHS menopause clinic in her area, but was told there was no budget. So, she started a private clinic, prescribing NHS-approved hormones, and it is now the biggest in the world, having gone from two doctors on its staff to 80 in three years, and still has a 8,000-patient waiting list. 'Every day I see women on their knees in here, desperate for the help they haven't received on the NHS. I'm not GP-bashing, but the need for education is desperate.'

Anyway, to cut to the happy ending, after a tiny bit of adjustment of the progesterone, my new prescription stopped all the bleeding. I was healthy at last – and now very worried about what was happening to other women out there in the menopause maze. I met another woman in the film industry who had suffered exactly the same compounds-to-cancer-tests experience as me. As I went into investigative-journalist mode, I was astounded at what Dr Newson told me about the neglect of menopause treatment. She told me about Janice Wilson (Chapter 2), who was given 12 sessions of electroconvulsive therapy instead of HRT, and about a survey of 3,000 menopausal patients, 66 per cent of whom were offered antidepressants instead of HRT.[13] And Dr Newson suggested I look up the latest warnings about compounded bioidentical HRT.

It turned out that the experts – the British Menopause Society and the Royal College of Obstetricians and Gynaecologists – had become so concerned by the increasing use of compounded HRT they had issued a statement of condemnation[14] – but your average googling patient, like me, probably won't find it. The NHS website also says vaguely, under 'Alternatives' to HRT, that compounded hormones 'are not regulated and it's not clear how safe they are'.[15] Obviously, some clinics have better reputations than others and use licensed pharmacies, but how would you find that out? I interviewed Haitham Hamoda, the chair of the BMS and a consultant gynaecologist at King's College Hospital, where 95 per cent of his menopausal patients are on NHS-regulated body-identical hormones. He said: 'Every expert in the field shares the same view and concerns about compounded hormones: they're unsafe, untested and unnecessary, and we're concerned about purity, potency and safety.'

So why are clinics still selling these compounds to patients? 'The hormones are supposedly compounded as one-offs for each individual, so they're not tested,' said Hamoda. The compounding pharmacies are usually registered with the General Pharmaceutical Council, but when you look into the regulations, they're about hygiene and whether medicines 'are obtained from a reputable source'.[16] The hormones themselves are probably obtained from a reputable source, but what do we know about the mixology? All cocktails are a little bit different, and how do you guard against that? Who you gonna call?

The clinics should be inspected by the Care Quality Commission,[17] which gives red, green and amber ratings. The Marion Gluck Clinic and the London Hormone Clinic were both passed as safe, effective and caring by the CQC. One of the questions the Commission asks is: 'Are medicines appropriately prescribed, administered and/or supplied to people in line with the relevant legislation, current national guidance or best available evidence?' But the CQC is underfunded and has a huge backlog of inspections. Hundreds of clinics are still dishing out lucrative unlicensed hormones to women and are not on the CQC's future-inspections list.

Women are vulnerable at this time in their lives, and hormones are often slipped into an expensive beauty package. I looked at the website of one clinic in Harley Street, which features a montage of abs and bums, and heavily emphasises the anti-ageing aspect of hormones. It also offers a 'Mommy Makeover' – a breast uplift, a tummy tuck and liposuction. 'At the center [sic] we want you to feel your best. Bioidentical hormone therapy . . . will be personalized for you by our highly educated and well-experienced doctor.' That scared me, just in terms of spelling and grammar. At time of writing, that well-experienced clinic was not on the CQC future-inspections list.

Yet many of the hormone clinics are not about beauty and Botox, and are staffed by menopause doctors so frustrated they leave the NHS to set up private practices offering compounded bioidenticals. I went to interview Dr Jan Toledano, who set up the London Hormone Clinic (LHC) after working as a specialist in women's health and genito-urinary medicine at London's St Bartholemew's Hospital for ten years. 'I was increasingly aware there was this large group of women who needed help, that didn't fit into any "women's problem" clinic. There was a black hole,' Toledo explained. I told her I wanted to know more about bioidentical compounded prescribing, and recounted my experience at the clinic I attended. (I wish I'd kept the lozenges, but I threw them away in a panic, so I can't have the hormone quantities in them tested to provide proof.) Such compounding problems are now causing disquiet in the industry. One of the London Hormone Clinic's pink Instagram posts says in large letters: 'LHC works with a registered pharmacy which has been compounding medicines for many years.'

Dr Toledano said she does use bioidentical lozenges and creams for some women. 'The compounding pharmacy I use is approved by the Medicines and Healthcare products Regulatory Agency and compounds for the NHS too.' Often, she offers women the NHS-approved preparations. 'But some women have allergies or can't tolerate micronised progesterone, so we need compounded bioidentical alternatives.'

Of my bad compounded batch, she said: 'There is never a reason to bleed like that. They should have done something straight away.'

I was fortunate that I stopped the compounded hormones before they did permanent damage to my uterus, but until NHS menopause care and doctors' knowledge of HRT prescription improves, desperate patients will try alternatives from unregulated sources. In my rush to escape an imaginary case of breast cancer, I ended up risking of a real case of uterine cancer.

My motivations were typical. A 2017 American survey titled 'Why women choose compounded bioidentical hormone therapy: lessons from a qualitative study of menopausal decision-making' showed that 35 per cent of HRT users chose the compounded version, and there were 'push motivations' that drove women away from conventional hormone therapy and alternative therapies, and 'pull motivations' that attracted women to compounded hormones.[18] The 'push motivations' were fear and uncertainty about the safety of conventional HRT and an aversion to horse-urine-derived estrogen, as well as 'overarching *distrust* of a medical system perceived as dismissive of their concerns and overly reliant on pharmaceuticals'. The 'pull motivations', towards compounded hormones, were that women believed them to be safer, tailored to their individual needs and 'accompanied by enhanced clinical care and attention'.

The compounded hormone market in America is vast compared with the UK (where there are hundreds of clinics but no official figures so far). A 2018 study estimated that of the 21 million annual prescriptions for natural progesterone in America, 18 million were compounded. According to another analysis, between 28 and 39 million individual hormone prescriptions per year are compounded, and an estimated 1–2.5 million US women over the age of 40 are currently using compounded hormones.[19] That same paper surveyed 3,000 women on compounded hormones and three quarters of them had no idea whether or not compounded hormones were approved by the US Food and Drug Administration (FDA). They're not. In fact, the FDA website says: 'Because compounded drugs are not FDA-approved, FDA does not verify their safety, effectiveness, or quality before they are marketed. In addition, poor compounding practices can result in serious drug quality problems, such as contamination or a drug that contains too much active ingredient. This can lead to serious patient injury and death.'[20]

Serious is an understatement. In 2012, a compounding pharmacy in Massachusetts sent out a bad batch of steroid injections contaminated with fungal meningitis that killed 64 people and caused over 600 more to become unwell. In 2018, during an FDA inspection of the large hormone-compounding company BioTE Medical, 'investigators uncovered information about 4,202 adverse events that had never been reported to the agency . . . hormone pellets were possibly associated with endometrial cancer, prostate cancer, strokes, heart attacks, deep vein thrombosis, cellulitis and pellet extrusion.'[21] The FDA is currently working with the National Academies of Sciences, Engineering, and Medicine to conduct a study on the risks associated with compounded hormones.

The American compounded HRT story is an investigation that could fill another book, but small pieces of work are targeting the issue already. In 2013, the America's Fund for Investigative Journalism and the UK's *More* magazine acquired 12 different samples of compounded hormones intended for menopausal women and tested them in a laboratory.[22] Even the simple business of weighing the supposedly 100mg hormone lozenges turned out to be revealing for the investigation – the heaviest weighed 102mg and the lightest 80mg. Worse still, the percentages of hormones were utterly out of whack in all 12 compound samples – some contained only 60 per cent of what was claimed.

Why is this omnishambles allowed to continue unregulated in America and the UK? Millions of women end up in this sector because the NHS in the UK and insurance companies in the USA are failing to provide safe services. And we are desperate – so desperate that when I look back on my incident and see that I continued to take the compounded HRT throughout the hospital tests, I am astonished. But I am even more astonished that it took a journalist, rather than three NHS doctors, to give me sensible advice.

You'll be glad to hear that my three friends who recommended bioidentical hormones to me have thrown away their private compounded prescriptions and are all on safer, NHS-approved hormones – although one keeps being sporadically refused HRT by her older, male GP. 'I need a letter from your ob-gyn to confirm this,' he said last time, grumpily sending her away. But she doesn't have an ob-gyn, and it's a GPs job to prescribe HRT. She has had to ask the practice for another doctor.

It's not just menopausal women who are struggling to know who to trust in the hormone market. Many men get top-ups of testosterone, and transgender people have turned to unofficial sources for years to get HRT. New findings show that 21 per cent of transgender Americans have had their request for HRT denied by insurance companies, and 9 per cent have used HRT from unlicensed sources.[23] There's no similar study in the UK, but dozens of private transgender hormone clinics have opened here in the past few years, some of which offer compounded hormones to patients who cannot get timely help on the NHS. Again, it's important for transgender people to know that NHS-approved natural hormones exist, and can still be privately prescribed.

Reading over this chapter, I still feel a strange sense of shame that my – how to put it? – my *addiction* to the life-repairing effects of HRT led me to cause all this unnecessary work for those hospital consultants; and that over a couple of years I handed over around £1,000 to fuel that dodgy addiction. When I was making the menopause documentary with Davina McCall, she talked about her feelings when first going on HRT privately (because she feared an NHS snub) and said the same thing: 'I was so full of shame about using HRT that I didn't go public for years.'

Why should we feel this shame? Some women who achieve some kind of natural menopausal nirvana condemn their weaker sisters or recoil from replacement hormones in horror. But as Dr Newson points out, 'no one is giving out any medals to women who soldier through menopause'. Indeed, some natural-menopause support groups may well become hip replacement support groups in later life. But I felt embarrassed for a long time, until I started studying the science and realised that the menopause was an inadequate description of a female hormone deficiency that will last the rest of your life. 'If your thyroid isn't working,' says Newson, 'do you say, "Oh, I'll soldier on without thyroxine?"'

Of course, women repair and rejuvenate their outsides all

the time, but that, too, has its secret club, where muffin tops are minimised, pouts are plumped, and brows are Botoxed, and no one says a word. So, how did something as important as our health for the second half of our lives end up being sold on the sly by unregulated beauty parlours?

Because it was ever thus. Indeed, women have brewed secret potions for other women's troubles since time began. I did, however, come across the first mention of the first compounded menopause medicine, made by Mrs Lydia Pinkham of Massachusetts in 1885. She created a somewhat alcoholic herbal potion that included black cohosh, fenugreek and unicorn root, which was supposed to relieve menopausal and menstrual symptoms. Mrs Pinkham provided a bespoke service, and her business saved her husband from bankruptcy. Wikipedia adds: 'Pinkham urged women to write to her personally, and she would maintain the correspondence in order to expose the customer to more persuasive claims for the remedy. Clearly the replies were not all written by Pinkham herself, as they continued after her death.'[24]

You may know the drinking song about Lydia Pinkham, also known as 'Lily the Pink'. And let it be a warning to you of quackery then and now:

> We'll drink a drink, a drink
> To Lily the Pink, the Pink, the Pink
> The saviour of the human race
> For she invented medicinal compound
> Most efficacious in every case!

10

THE MENOPAUSE AND BREAST CANCER

Researching this chapter, I started thinking about my own breasts, and our long, difficult and occasionally rewarding journey together since they popped up over 40 years ago. It is clear to me that, unlike most other, more reliable, parts of the body, breasts have a mind of their own. You have no idea what they'll do next. They're at their glorious best during sex, a higher power calling on a direct line to your clitoris and vagina. They're at their worst just before a period, a bag of marbles delivering a heavy, dull ache and an occasional mean-girl stab. They're possessed a few weeks after you get pregnant, improbably expanding like two stone grapefruits. They're a miracle fount of pulsating, thought-controlled milk at childbirth, gashed by cracked nipples. And later in life they're a lurking presence, an unpredictable source of fear and joy. Is that a pea-sized lump I feel in the shower? And will it go away after my period?

As you approach menopause, your breasts tend to get less

bodacious. Your milk system shuts down for good, and tissue in your breast shrinks. The skin gets less elastic and begins to sag – less so if you're topping up your estrogen. There is an upside, though. I found that after my periods stopped the 28-day cycle of lumps and pain went away along with the lunar insanity of breast tissue, and at last my breasts were soft and predictable. However, the perimenopause and menopause are the times when the medical system starts taking a suspicious interest in our breasts, since breast cancer rates roughly double when you hit aged 45,[1] and keep on growing. No one seems to know exactly why.

One in seven women will get breast cancer.[3] It hangs over women like a malevolent pall. No other affliction seems to have the same visceral terror for women (and men), cutting into the very essence of womanhood and motherhood. By the time you're in your fifties, like me, breast cancer will be an insidious addition to your wider friendship group. Five of my girlfriends have had it. Four have recovered, and one has died. It's inevitable. It's fucked up.

Our breasts move in mysterious ways, and their secrets can only be revealed when crushed in the Perspex vice of a mammogram machine. I don't blame the operators, who have to knead and compress the tissue as gently as they can, as you lean forward, naked from the waist up, waiting for your previously round breast to be turned into a pancake. I know the breast needs to be held still for a clear image. I just wish Patrick Panetta and Jack Wennet, the inventors of the mammogram machine, had breasts themselves, so they knew how painful and humiliating the experience is. Perhaps with this in mind, one of my favourite film directors, Nicole Holofcener, featured mammogram after mammogram to a jaunty tune in the opening sequence of her comedy *Please Give*. Rebecca Hall played the mammogram technician, and the breasts played themselves – all shapes and sizes, mostly vintage.

Nowadays, eight out of ten women diagnosed with breast cancer are predicted to survive their disease for at least ten years,[4] so living healthily after recovery is incredibly important, and we will go on to discuss the surprising role that body-identical HRT can have post-cancer. In fact, the leading cause of death for women in the UK is not breast cancer at all, which comes in at number seven in the mortality top ten. Women are most likely to die of Alzheimer's disease and dementia, followed by heart disease and lung cancer. So what's the main risk, aside from gender and genetic factors, for breast cancer? 'Age,' replies oncologist Michael Baum. 'Women in their sixties and seventies are the biggest group.' Being obese is also a warning sign – it *doubles* your chances of getting breast cancer – and having a mutation in the tumour-suppressing BRCA1 or BRCA2 genes increases your chances of cancer by the age of 70 to around 65 per cent.[5] But much less than 1 per cent of the population has those genes.[6] Baum is Professor Emeritus of Surgery and visiting Professor of Medical Humanities at University College London, and believes the use of HRT is but a hormonal drop in the water as a cancer risk compared with genetics, age, obesity or smoking. A British Menopause Society summary of studies put the added cancer risk from HRT in the key 50–59 age group at an extra 4 in 1,000 women over five years' use,[7] but even without HRT around 23 out of 1,000 women of that age get breast cancer. Again, it's worth emphasising that is the risk from the older, combined, synthetic pills. But most women are basing their decision on emotions, not health statistics, and they are still freaked out by any risk at all.

I've had a lot of mammograms. If you have dense breast tissue (the aforementioned bag of marbles), it's hard to see what's going on in there. A few years ago, when I still had my periods, I found a grape-sized lump in my breast, and the mammogram looked dodgy so I was sent to a consultant for an ultrasound. Most of us know that nauseating, grinding, sleep-stealing fear that you keep to yourself while waiting for weeks for investigation, because there's no point in making a fuss – yet. In fact, the lump was benign, filled with liquid, and the doctor cheerily syringed it out. 'That's my favourite moment in this job,' says Professor Baum. 'A woman comes in worried about cancer, and in a moment, it's magically gone.' More recently, my mammogram showed a sprinkle of calcium deposits, and I had to have a biopsy. I thought that was going to be a small affair, but a burly nurse held me down while a doctor armed with a core-needle biopsy tool – more like a spring-loaded no. 2 knitting needle – stabbed my chest while peering at a screen. My breast was swollen and purple with bruising for weeks afterwards, but a month later I got the all clear.

These minor brushes with the distant possibility of breast cancer can never give one a sense of the violation, loss and agony involved in a lumpectomy or a mastectomy followed by chemotherapy and radiotherapy. I remember visiting one of my friends in hospital after her mastectomy, and she was massively brave, a tube draining liquid at one side, the newly flat side casually covered by a flowing purple silk scarf. I just wanted to cry, but she was tougher than that and talked politics as usual. I also met author and family mediator Kate Figes, who later died of triple-negative breast cancer, aged 62. She invited me round for tea in her kitchen and gave me funny, wise advice about divorce and moving on just when I needed it, but soon after she was diagnosed with cancer that had gone undetected in routine mammograms. 'Cancer is sneaky,' she said. 'There's no pain until it's too late. Cancer magnifies all of the anxieties, regrets and losses of midlife into one big horrifying goldfish bowl. It forces you to look back over your shoulder at the choices you have made, one last time.' Figes' last book, *On Smaller Dogs and Larger Life Questions*, charts the journey through midlife – in her case with her family and Zeus, a wire-haired dachshund.

The crosshairs of science and art keep meeting as I write this book. Professor Baum has tracked breast cancer in art and literature back to the Egyptians,[8] and for scientific reasons is fascinated by Rembrandt's painting *Bathsheba at her Bath*, an exquisite, russet-haired, glowing nude from 1654. In the Hebrew Bible, Bathsheba was already married, but was 'summoned' by King David, after he saw her bathing and lusted after her. Eventually, she gave birth to their son Solomon. But Rembrandt's work is less about lust and more about tender, domestic adoration: his Bathsheba is Hendrickje Stoffels, his partner, housekeeper and muse. Eventually, she gave birth to their daughter. The Old Master captured his young mistress in intimate and forensic detail: her glinting pearl-drop earrings, her pensive look, her voluptuous stomach, and her neat, round breasts, one bearing a slight bruised shadow and puckering. Had Rembrandt inadvertently painted one of the earliest depictions of breast cancer? 'You can see the dimple on the upper outer quadrant of her left breast,' writes Baum of the painting, which now hangs in the Louvre. 'Hendrickje Stoffels died nine years after this painting, and the record of her illness and dying was very characteristic of a woman with advanced breast cancer with secondaries [metastasis] to the liver.'

Baum is a maverick genius as well as a massive figure in the improvement of breast cancer care in the UK, encouraging the use of lumpectomy rather than radical mastectomy, chairing the largest trial in the world comparing the relative benefits of tamoxifen with another drug in the management of breast cancer. He also pioneered the use of intraoperative radiotherapy at the time of lumpectomy, giving one killer blast of radiation to the tumour bed in the operating theatre, rather than asking women to come every day for six miserable weeks of radiotherapy. (After learning that women in rural India were unable to travel to a city hospital every day for radiotherapy, he helped find this smart solution.) Professor Baum's mother died of breast cancer, and he remembers the 'madness of the cure', the brutality of the old-fashioned chemotherapy, and her long black hair falling out. Thus, he very much believes in balancing women's cancer treatment with their quality of life: 'Women are much more than the sum of their two breasts.'

More controversially, Professor Baum is among a small but growing group of oncologists who have prescribed HRT to some breast cancer survivors after a good recovery from a lumpectomy or mastectomy. More than most people, Professor Baum has sat talking to women about their hopes for the future after mastectomy, and he has also studied the research linking the older forms of HRT to slight increases in breast cancer rates. He believes the Women's Health Initiative study has damaged women's health irreparably. 'I will never forgive them for what they've done – it's a sorry, sad story.' He considers the risks from body-identical HRT to be low and is hopeful of a better outcome. 'Left to me, for women with menopausal symptoms, with or without their uterus, the benefits of hormone replacement outweigh the hazards.' His wife Judy took HRT for seven years, and he advised his daughter, Katie Taylor, who runs the Latte Lounge[9] support group for midlife women, to start body-identical regulated HRT when she was perimenopausal.

But offering HRT to breast cancer survivors with debilitating menopausal symptoms is a bigger step, and seems counterintuitive, as most breast cancers are estrogen- or progesterone-receptor positive. (A cancer is called estrogen-receptor-positive if it has receptors for estrogen. This suggests that the cancer cells, like normal breast cells, may receive signals from estrogen or progesterone that could promote their growth.) But it turns out HRT in tandem with the anti-cancer drug tamoxifen seems to work for some postmenopausal women who find their quality of life is unbearable on powerful aromatase-inhibitors like letrozole, which are given after cancer to completely block the body's own production of estrogen and can cause a perfect storm of menopausal symptoms.[10]

Some published reports have found that abnormal estrogen levels increase the chance of a woman developing breast cancer.[11] But Professor Baum explains that the simplistic view, that 'estrogen equals breast cancer', is wrong. It's far, far more complicated and subtle than that. 'If estrogen caused breast cancer then premenopausal women would have more cancers than postmenopausal women. Pregnant women with high estrogen levels have better breast cancer recovery rates, and it's no surprise to me that women on long-term estrogen-only HRT have a lower rate of breast cancer,' says Professor Baum, referring to the other arm of the 18-year WHI study, which investigated women on estrogen-only HRT, who had a 23 per cent lower rate of breast cancer than those on a placebo.[12] That good news was seriously under-reported at the time.

Tamoxifen, which has changed the outcomes of so many breast cancer survivors for the better, actually has an estrogen-like effect. 'We still don't know quite how it works,' says Professor Baum, 'but we do know it can slightly increase the risk of endometrial cancer, which is proof it's estrogenic.' So, if estrogen is not the initial cause of cancer, once the tumour has been removed and all the cancer cells zapped, is it safe for breast cancer survivors to take HRT? And if estrogen is not the culprit, was there something in the synthetic progestins of the old kind of combination oral HRT that helped to cause cancer, as suggested in the previous chapter? Thanks to good old medical sexism, very little research into this has been funded so far, but the question is going mainstream: the debate at the 2021 British Menopause Society conference was 'This house believes that HRT can be taken by women living with breast cancer.'

Midlife women want the answers now, not in ten or twenty years. Cancer survivors want to live a full life, not a half life, and the effect of estrogen depletion from aromatase-inhibitor drugs can be hell. This was the case for my friend Kirsty Lang, a broadcaster and journalist who has made a determined march through breast cancer, with just one month off work. We met over 20 years ago, in Paris, when she was the correspondent there for the *Sunday Times* and I was a columnist for *The Times*. Since then, she has presented BBC Radio 4's *Front Row* for over a decade. I remember Lang downplaying her diagnosis four years ago, when she was 53, and sounding resolutely cheerful on the phone. 'I'm going to get a proper wig, in case all my hair falls out from chemo,' she said before the operation. She felt that her job as a freelance presenter needed her to be conventionally presentable; no scarves or hats. Such are the expectations upon women, even when they are seriously ill. 'When I think about breast cancer, I have an image of an evil Greek god wanting to take revenge on womankind: "Not only am I going to give you cancer, but I'm going to remove all signs of your femininity. I'm going to chop your breasts off and make you lose your hair!"'

There's not much we can do about surgery, but there is help on the hair front. 'Do you want someone to come with you to the wig place?' I asked tentatively. She accepted my offer, so one afternoon we ended up in a strange basement salon in London's Wimpole Street, and Lang, who has a red bob in a similar shade to Bathsheba, sat in front of a mirror trying on real-hair wigs that would be styled to suit her. One wig was terrific, a perfect match. 'You look like Julianne Moore!' I said, taking some photographs. For added convenience, the wig seemed to stay permanently coiffed and blow-dried.

Then came the hard stuff. Lang's breast lump was tiny, only discovered in a routine mammogram, but it was a grade 3 cancer: 'which meant it was growing fast and on the move', recalled Lang. As the consultant scheduled a lumpectomy, the first thing Lang asked was: 'Oh my god – is it my fault, because I'm taking HRT?' She had been happily on HRT for nearly five years, since she was 48. The surgeon said: 'Probably not; more likely it's family history or lifestyle factors.' He cited maybe alcohol, or the fact that she had once been a smoker, plus Lang's maternal grandmother had died of breast cancer in her fifties. 'But he did say, because it was an estrogen-sensitive cancer, my HRT might have acted like a sort of "fertiliser" on the tumour. Fertiliser! I was horrified,' she remembers. She went home and threw all her HRT patches in the bin.

Lang was scheduled for a lumpectomy and six weeks of radiotherapy but, being on a freelance contract at the BBC, she didn't get any sick pay, so six weeks off was a problem. A friend told her about the alternative of a one-off shot of radiation during the operation – but there were only six NHS machines in the UK, a hopeless postcode lottery. 'My lump was on my left breast, and your heart is more towards that side, so I didn't like the idea of radiation being beamed over my heart every day,' says Lang. Indeed, breast cancer survivors have a higher rate of death from heart disease, perhaps due to radiation as well as lack of estrogen.[13] Lang found there was an intraoperative radiation machine in Swindon, and luckily the BBC's health insurance paid. 'I left hospital that night and was back at work within a week, with no side effects.' Chemotherapy was tougher, but she didn't feel too sick and went on Fridays so she could recover over the weekend.

How many breast cancer survivors lose their jobs or give up working as breast cancer and the menopause strike at the same time? Following her own experience, Lang spoke out at the Digital, Culture, Media and Sport Select Committee in March 2018, which was investigating why the BBC had made staff members go freelance for tax purposes. She talked about working through cancer to keep her contract. 'I speak for many people in this situation,' she told the committee. 'I have seen many women presenters being deprived of maternity leave, I have seen many colleagues being deprived of sick pay, and we keep on doing it because we love the job.'

Her struggle didn't end there. After surgery, Lang was put on the aromatase-inhibitor letrozole, 'which hoovers up every bit of your estrogen. I could feel it drying me up.' Within a few weeks, the original menopausal symptoms she'd had before HRT came back. 'But this time, they were turbocharged. Whereas, before, I would get the occasional hot flush, I was now getting one or two an hour, day and night. I was dripping with sweat. I've had to change my entire wardrobe over the last three years. I can't wear any synthetic materials, and I always have to wear layers of clothes. I often changed my shirt at the office because it was drenched in sweat. It was really hard.' Her sleep was terrible. But the worst symptom was the stiffness in her joints. 'I was crawling out of bed in the morning like a little old lady, with my hands like claws. Feet hurting, knees hurting.'

Her sex life was ruined by vaginal dryness. She also began to get urinary tract infections. Fortunately, her oncologist gave her vaginal estrogen cream and pessaries to deal with the dryness, and the topical dose is tiny – the equivalent in a year to one or two HRT pills – so it's considered safe even for cancer survivors.[14] Within weeks she felt better and the dryness went away. Lang battled on with letrozole for two years, but her quality of life was really low. She tried giving up alcohol and coffee, which helped a tiny bit with the flushes, 'but I needed *some* tiny pleasures'. She also tried an antidepressant for a few weeks, 'but I was so nauseous and bombed out, I thought I'd rather have the hot flushes back.'

Every woman is different, and some do much better on aromatase-inhibitors like letrozole. My friend Vanora Bennett, who is a novelist and journalist, has been on letrozole for two years. She went through the menopause before her cancer was diagnosed, and does not have hot flushes – just occasional sleeplessness (which we successfully experimented on with CBD oil capsules – see Chapter 7). But aromatase-inhibitors are dastardly, adding to natural postmenopausal loss of bone density. 'I went for a DEXA scan and they told me I had osteoporosis in my spine,' said Bennett. She is carrying on with the drug, but is now on anti-osteoporosis medication too. (Dr Louise Newson has written a very useful booklet on strategies for coping with menopause symptoms after breast cancer.[15])

Lang, too, was worried about osteoporosis, but she always assumed that going back on HRT was not an option. Then she was asked to chair a conference of breast cancer experts for the Royal Society, where she attended a lecture by the American oncologist Professor Avrum Bluming. 'I was spellbound by what this man was saying. He had breast cancer patients on HRT, including his own wife and daughter.' He argued that a review of research round the world, including his own 14-year study, found that most women with successfully treated breast cancer can take HRT without an increased risk of recurrence.[16]

I interviewed Professor Bluming, who lives in California and is the author of *Estrogen Matters* with Carol Tavris, and he said that women are told: '"You've survived breast cancer – why aren't you happy?",' adding, 'One of those women happened to be my wife.' In the book, he wondered why he would ever consider giving HRT to women with a history of breast cancer. 'What if the cancer returned? What if I were responsible for the death of a patient who, without my well-intentioned help, would have remained cured?'[17] But he was encouraged by the work of other oncologists, including Professor Michael Baum. Professor Bluming got permission from the US Food and Drugs Administration to start a trial. (Interestingly, there was no placebo in the trial, because Bluming was aware that women usually know whether they on genuine HRT as their hot flushes subside within days.) His trial was small, but a later meta-analysis of 15 similar studies showed a 10 per cent lower rate of breast cancer recurrence compared with no treatment.[18] However, the Swedish HABITS (HRT After Breast Cancer – Is It Safe?)[19] trial in 2004 was stopped early due to an increased risk of recurrence following treatment of breast cancer, which was eventually attributed to higher progestin exposure,[20] as the study used synthetic, not body-identical HRT.

Lang went to see her oncologist, who said, 'Oh yes, I do have a small cohort of women on HRT, but their quality of life was so terrible without it.' He had never mentioned HRT was a possibility. 'You don't seem to be suffering too much,' he added. 'If you can stand letrozole, I would put up with it.' Lang's quality of life was awful – those claw hands stay most in my mind – but even her friends and colleagues had no idea exactly what she was going through. She really played it down, as so many women do. But she investigated the science, listened to experts, and decided to try HRT again. Her oncologist agreed to change her over to tamoxifen, which is compatible with HRT and is almost as protective as letrozole. (There's an interesting *Lancet* paper on taking letrozole and later tamoxifen.[21]) 'This is not for everybody. This is all about one's capacity and propensity to take risks,' said Lang, who has remained on HRT.

At the same time, once her symptoms had been dissipated by HRT, Lang had the strength to have a holistic overhaul, and now makes sure she has days off alcohol every week and takes much more exercise. 'I'm getting off the Tube a couple of stops early,' she says. For one of the most astonishing statistics around breast cancer survivors (and you know by now how much I like a good statistic) is that women who take brisk exercise for 30 minutes a day, five days a week, lower their chances of breast cancer recurring by 40 per cent.[22] That's huge. That's what doctors and the media should be talking about. Conversely, women who gain more than 10 per cent in weight after diagnosis have an increased risk of dying.[23] After cancer, eating well and exercising are not just lifestyle choices, like wearing something more fashionable; they are survival choices. Cognitive behavioural therapy (CBT) also seems to reduce 'overwhelming' menopausal symptoms for breast cancer survivors not using HRT. Research led by Swansea University found that women who received six weeks of group CBT from a breast-care nurse reported that their menopausal symptoms, such as such as hot flushes and night sweats, became significantly less distressing, and reduced by 28 per cent.[24]

Feeling motivated enough to stay mentally and physically healthy after cancer is really important, but that's clearly not what's happening, and this is where thinking about using body-identical HRT is key. An American study of 750,000 breast cancer survivors showed that, compared with women in the general population, they were 37 per cent more likely to commit suicide.[25] Dr Charlotte Fleming, a consultant gynaecologist who set up the first specialist menopause clinic in Wales, increasingly focuses on helping long-term breast cancer survivors. 'When estrogen levels are undetectable, women feel absolutely ghastly. People come to me saying, "I can't live like this. I have suicidal plans. I would rather have a second breast cancer than live like this",' explains Fleming. 'A woman lives in her own skin twenty-four hours a day and she chooses the risks she takes.' Fleming says few people in the UK are even prepared to discuss HRT after breast cancer, 'but I'm in favour of giving women their own choices. There are the women who say, "Blow it, I want to be able to have sex."'

Bluming, Baum and Fleming are at a mature stage in their careers, where they can afford to question the status quo. But many brilliant oncologists on the frontline are still on the fence on this subject. 'HRT after breast cancer?' said Tony Howell, who is Chair in Breast Oncology at Manchester University and Professor of Medical Oncology at the Christie Hospital. 'That's a tricky one. Women aren't average-risk – half have a lower risk and half have a higher risk. There are so many variables.' And not everyone will try to improve those variables by taking the wellness precautions that Lang did. Frankly, it's hard enough for women to make these life-altering decisions, so it would be great if doctors were on the case, but there's a huge crevasse in medical education. The breast cancer survivors who seek out help and information are middle-class, the same as those women who seek out the best HRT. Most NHS oncologists would never bring up the subject of post-cancer

HRT, and the majority instead opt for the apparently safe option of advising distraught women to take antidepressants. Patients need more choice and information.

Perhaps the best known example of informed patient choice is the decision by the American actress Angelina Jolie in 2013 to have a preventative double mastectomy and her ovaries and fallopian tubes removed after she found she had the BRCA1 tumour-suppressing-gene mutation. This procedure is available on the NHS too, and the Royal Marsden Hospital in London says that afterwards the cancer risk is reduced by around 90 per cent.[26] In her *New York Times*, 'Diary of a Surgery' Jolie wrote that having the gene put her at an '87 per cent risk of breast cancer and a 50 per cent risk of ovarian cancer, although the risk is different in the case of each woman. Once I knew that this was my reality, I decided to be proactive and to minimize the risk as much as I could.'[27] Jolie's mother died aged 56 after a ten-year struggle with ovarian cancer.

After the removal of her ovaries, Jolie explained she went into early menopause aged 39. She began taking HRT: 'I have a little clear patch that contains bioidentical estrogen. A progesterone IUD was inserted in my uterus. It will help me maintain a hormonal balance, but more important it will help prevent uterine cancer. I chose to keep my uterus because cancer in that location is not part of my family history.' A British Menopause Society statement said that replacing estrogen with HRT was safe after removal of the ovaries.[28] Jolie added that she feels, 'feminine and grounded in the choices I am making for myself'. Following her operations, she directed three films, starred in the Disney sequel to *Maleficent* and voiced Master Tigress in *Kung Fu Panda 3*. That's recovery for you.

While the world was shocked by Jolie's decision, at first, Professor Baum was not. 'Those are mutations of very powerful genes, with a chance of breast cancer of the aggressive type. I must reluctantly agree that a bilateral mastectomy was a sensible choice. There's good evidence. Angelina Jolie is brilliant – what a courageous woman. In future we must do better than surgery. Surely soon there will be molecular correction for cases like Jolie's.' This is about repairing or changing the sequence of DNA in cells, but science has a long way to go, and so far this has only been tested in the laboratory.[29]

It's scary how easy it is to find out if you have the BRCA1 mutation, from a test on the NHS (if you have a family history) or privately. When my son gave me a £79 ancestry test from 23andMe, one of the popular DNA testing services, I discovered that you can also get a 'Health and Ancestry' test for £149,[30] which will give you a 'predisposition report' on the BRCA gene mutations and on the APOE4 gene, which is a possible indicator for Alzheimer's. I don't want to know whether I have the Alzheimer's gene, and I was not at all surprised when my DNA came back as basically potato-based Scottish and Irish. But what should women do if they test positive for the BRCA mutation? Wait and see? Eat Pray Love? Copy Angelina Jolie? Or hope science will speed up and come to their rescue?

The positive choices of women like Jolie and Lang are inspiring – and frightening – for all of us staring into this mammary wheel of fortune. But I can report back that Lang has been cancer-free for six years since her operation, and has enjoyed life on HRT for the past four.

Last but not least, what happened to our first breast cancer patient, Hendrickje Stoffels? In 1654, as well as posing nude, she gave birth to Rembrandt's daughter, Cornelia, and the couple lived together until Stoffels died in 1663. They remained unwed, much to the irritation of the Reformed Church, who summoned Stoffels several times until she confessed her sin: she had 'stained herself by fornication with Rembrandt'.[31] But it seems that Stoffels was not bothered by her sins or her lurking breast tumour for years. In fact, she became Rembrandt's business manager after he went bankrupt (he was hopeless with money) and opened an art shop with Titus, the painter's son from his earlier marriage, where she sold her lover's paintings. And here's the best bit: in order to protect Rembrandt from money lenders, Stoffels and Titus became his employers.[32] So Stoffels was actually Rembrandt's boss, her support probably facilitating his burst of productivity in the early 1660s. As Professor Baum would say, a woman is more than the sum of her two breasts.

11

DO HORMONES HELP PREVENT ALZHEIMER'S DISEASE?

What's the biggest killer of women? Heart disease? Pneumonia? Lung cancer? Breast cancer? No. The top female serial killer in the UK is Alzheimer's disease and dementia, a lingering death of the mind. We don't want to think about it. Not now, not ever. But it is the future for one in five women, and one in eleven men[1] – probably someone you know.

My paternal grandfather, Alexander Caldwell Muir, had Alzheimer's. He died before I was born, but he lived with my mum and dad in his final years. Photographs from that time show a lanky, besuited figure (he'd run a drapery and hat shop in Glasgow), a man in good health – except for the fact he became convinced my dad, his only son, was actually the lodger, and would whisper his dark suspicions about the stranger in the flat to my mum. This story was told affectionately, as eccentric family lore, but I now realise my mother, Ella, knew about living with dementia long before she was diagnosed with it herself. She died eight years ago after a long haul through Alzheimer's disease and I am uneasily aware that could be the inheritance for me, and eventually my daughter.

I've always paid attention to Alzheimer's research in the news, from the day my once rapier-sharp mum first went for a dementia test with her lovely GP in Glasgow. Smart as ever, Ella wore a jacket from the Jaeger sale, little heels, and carried her good leather handbag for the appointment. Dignity mattered. We didn't really discuss what was happening as we walked there; my mum felt sure her GP would sort it out – she'd been brilliant when my dad fought through a series of strokes before he died. The interview in the surgery was torture: humiliation for my mother, and agony for me sitting listening, as the doctor gently asked: 'Who is the prime minister?', 'What's your date of birth?' and 'What was the name of your school?' Ella knew the prime minister (and had quite a low opinion of him), but she was vague and tried to cover up on the school front. The season might have been autumn or spring; she wasn't entirely sure. She faltered counting backwards and remembering a short shopping list. What were my mother's feelings? She didn't answer that question either.

Ella was in her early eighties and still living independently then. She was well enough to know what was happening, so the NHS memory clinic in Drumchapel suggested she took a drug that prevents the breakdown of the brain chemical acetylcholine and was supposed to result in a small benefit in mental function, though it does not halt the disease. It just gave her awful nausea – and inevitably she forgot to take the tablets unless prompted by a visiting carer, so eventually we gave up. Later, she must have been aware of how fast her memories were disappearing, and how the new ones failed to stick. Having been a woman who never took more than a wee sherry or a gin and tonic after 6 p.m., for two awful years she began drinking all day to forget. She had a couple of nasty falls. Then she eventually forgot to drink. We crashed in and out of crises, hospitals and eventually a care home. *There is no hope, there is no solution*, I thought. Two thirds of Alzheimer's patients are women, so what makes us so special, so unlucky? Then a surprising answer came, four years after Ella's death, as a by-product of the work I had started on the menopause. I discovered research on how important hormones are to brain function.

Increasingly, experts like Professor Philip Sarrel at Yale University are saying that hot flushes are 'the canary in the coal mine',[2] a warning sign of the damage to come as we age, particularly when it comes to our brains. The more hot flushes we suffer, the more our cognitive decline in the short term,[3] and in the long term it turns out that HRT is a no-brainer for those who want to protect their brainpower.[4]

Reading up on estrogen's and testosterone's effect on cognitive function and memory loss around menopause was revelatory. I came upon the work of two extraordinary American women and interviewed them both: Dr Roberta Diaz Brinton, director of the Center for Innovation in Brain Science at the University of Arizona and Dr Lisa Mosconi of the Weill Cornell Women's Brain Initiative and author of *The XX Brain: The Groundbreaking Science Empowering Women to Maximise Cognitive Health and Prevent Alzheimer's Disease*.[5] 'Until now, medical research has focused on "bikini medicine", assuming that women are essentially men with breasts and tubes,' said Mosconi. 'We need to recognise that women's brains age distinctly from men's, due mostly to the decline of a key brain-protective hormone: estrogen.'

This area of research may change the future for millions of women at risk. But before we hear the good news, let's start with something scary, because the first thing I saw when I went on Mosconi's website was two PET scans, of a premenopausal and postmenopausal brain, *in a normal woman*, not one with dementia. The postmenopausal brain had far less activity; the colours were clearly dimmer.[6] I called Mosconi and she explained: 'The brighter the colour on the brain scan, the more the activity, and the postmenopausal woman's brain is darker and the activity is thirty per cent less.' Thirty per cent? Could that be true? Mosconi said that might not happen to every woman at the same level – some just lose 20 per cent of activity, some even less – but this postmenopausal brain on the scan was still 'cognitively normal'.

After menopause, we are deprived of estrogen, and not always firing on all cylinders, as estrogen regulates the transport of glucose, which is fuel for the brain.[7] 'The lack of fuel explains why women experience they are off their game,' explained Dr Roberta Diaz Brinton. 'They can play the game, just not as well.'

Dr Mosconi pointed to the bodily signs that herald turmoil in the mind: 'When skin wrinkles, bones get frail, and hair dries and thins after menopause, the lack of estrogen has a similar effect on our brains, weakening our neurons.' She is also a daughter of Alzheimer's. Mosconi's father was diagnosed in 2003 and died in 2011, and that difficult time 'propelled me to make it my mission to find a cure for this devastating illness', she says in the introduction to her book. She came to focus particularly on women, because of their higher rate of Alzheimer's, realising the longer a woman was fertile, the less chance she had of getting the disease. Losing estrogen at any time of life tips women into the 'at risk' bracket for dementia. Women who have early hysterectomies or oophorectomies (ovary removal) before the age of 50 have a greatly increased risk of early onset dementia due to the lack of estrogen.[8] Dr Brinton explained: 'Women who have had their ovaries removed before natural menopause show a deficit in short-term memory, long-term memory and logical reasoning. There's an increased risk of cognitive impairment or dementia and Parkinson's disease. The more estrogen a woman is exposed to in her lifetime, the better her brain fares.'

In 2021, some months after first I talked to Mosconi, she, Brinton and a number of other academics published an extraordinary study in the journal *Nature* of more than 160 women's brains in premenopause, perimenopause and postmenopause, looking at structure, blood flow and metabolism, as well as conducting memory and cognition tests.[9] Most of the women were not on HRT. The scientists compared the three stages of what was happening to women's brains with men of the same age, checked them out two years later, and the result was proof that female 'brain fog' is not imaginary, particularly in perimenopause. The brain scans showed that during the menopausal transition, women experienced a loss of grey matter – the brain cells that process information – and white matter – the connections between those cells. But in the postmenopausal brain that loss stopped, and in some cases brain volume then increased, though not to its premenopausal size. Just as it does before and after pregnancy, for most women the brain reboots after menopause. The scans showed that grey matter dips but then sometimes rises again, though white matter remains low, post-menopause. Most women seem to make up for this by increasing blood flow to the brain, but in some instances, however, compensatory responses are diminished or lacking. In an interview with the *New York Times* Mosconi said, 'What we found in women and not in men is that the brain changes quite a lot. The transition of menopause really leads to a whole remodelling.'[10] It's not great news for feminism and equality, which is perhaps why no one is shouting the news about these and similar studies from the rooftops, but it is also clear that most women manage the transition and slight loss, perhaps because we are more verbally deft than men.

More worryingly, Mosconi found that women who carried the APOE4 gene, which increases the chances of getting Alzheimer's disease, began to develop amyloid plaques, a sign of the disease, during perimenopause. 'We realised that cognitive decline was beginning for women in their forties and fifties, and that the window for therapeutic intervention was much earlier than we thought,' Mosconi said.

In a useful lecture for laypeople like us, which you can watch on YouTube, Brinton said: 'The brain is an energy hog. The brain is a Hummer, and the rest of the body is a Prius.'[11] She explained that the brain relies on blood flow for energy and about a third of the brain is made up of blood vessels. Estrogen helps open up the blood vessels and increases the levels of neurotransmitters like serotonin and dopamine.[12] When the brain runs out of fuel, it sends out a signal that it's starving, and at the moment, in some women, the brain can start to cannibalise itself.[13] 'Eventually the menopausal brain begins ransacking its own myelin, which surrounds nerves cells, to obtain enough ketone bodies [fatty acids] to work,' said Brinton. The breakdown of the myelin contributes to the amyloid plaques that clog up the brain during Alzheimer's. It's like getting limescale deposits inside a kettle, which eventually block the flow.

Alzheimer's shrinks the brain at about 400 per cent the rate of normal ageing.[14] Professor Ruth McKernan, a neuroscientist and trustee of Alzheimer's Research UK who works on new research projects with the Dementia Discovery Fund, told me: 'A brain with Alzheimer's loses about the weight of an orange compared to a healthy brain.' She thinks the role of estrogen is important, but that it is just one of the many factors. High blood pressure, which also increases after menopause, is another risk factor for dementia. But the loss of estrogen, which causes night sweats and anxiety, is significant because it causes fragmented sleep patterns. 'Slow-wave sleep improves the clearance of toxic waste in the brain. That's when we consolidate memories,' said McKernan. 'Women who have very bad hot flushes don't get much slow-wave sleep.' Basically, the brain's bin is filling up all day and no one is putting out the recycling at night. When you give menopausal women a sleep-tracking app or a Fitbit to wear at night, night sweats and heart palpitations cause their sleep patterns to be spiked with almost hourly awakenings, and only light or REM sleep. Long periods of deep, restorative, slow-wave sleep are sorely lacking. After taking HRT, however, sleep patterns almost always improve.[15]

There is a clear correlation between sleep quality and accumulation of amyloid plaques,[16] which cause Alzheimer's over the years. In particular, studies suggest that fragmented sleep and lower volumes of non-REM, slow-wave sleep may signal the greatest increases in amyloid plaque build-up.[17] So anything that increases your hours of deep sleep is a form of protection against Alzheimer's and dementia.

Those with night sweats and memory problems might want to pay attention now and try to mitigate these symptoms' later adverse effects by leading a healthier life in terms of diet and exercise, and considering some kind of estrogen-based therapy. Dr Mosconi recommends a Mediterranean diet for brain fuel, detailed in her book. 'You have three chances per day to feed your brain with nourishing foods or feed your brain foods that will negatively impact brain function and cognition,' she writes. Dropping red meats, sugar and saturated fats and replacing them with vegetables, fruit and lean protein, particularly oily fish, is the way forward. (There's another unsettling brain scan in Mosconi's research showing lower mental activity in a person on an unhealthy Western diet.[18]) She says that antioxidants like vitamin C, vitamin E and beta-carotene are important, as are polyunsaturated fatty acids like omega-3 and fibre. Mosconi also points out that chronic stress is associated with poor cognitive performance, and mindful mediation or yoga may help, as well as exercise. 'Exercise has been shown to be a strong preventative tool against Alzheimer's for men and women, but seems to be even more important for women.'[19]

The dangers are worse for those with the Alzheimer's APOE4 gene, which is usually – but not always – a predictor of trouble ahead. Dr Brinton points out that, aside from the rarer, early onset Alzheimer's, most women start to show signs of the disease in their seventies, 'but mood disturbances, insomnia and depression before that tell us the brain's circuits are changing.' The early signs and symptoms or prodromal phase of Alzheimer's is 20 years, 'and that takes us back with some pretty simple math to about fifty-one, the average age of menopause.'

This timing of the arrival of Alzheimer's symptoms makes sense when I consider my mother. I vaguely remember Ella having some hot flushes in her fifties, but she never made a fuss about them. Her brain was still revving in her sixties; she went to Bearsden Library every week, and eventually decided to stop reading fiction because she'd 'heard it all before', and moved into weighty biography. It was only in her early seventies that she began to repeat stories and questions, but I shrugged that off as normal. Later, she couldn't concentrate on books and became increasingly anxious, pacing around, keeping everything in its designated place. You didn't dare move a photograph on the sideboard. I put all that down to the stress she was under looking after my father, who had a series of small, disabling strokes and ended up with vascular dementia in a nursing home. When he died, Ella lost purpose, and the memory holes and lapses she had been covering up for years with conviction, energy and a large vocabulary suddenly stood out in frightening relief.

But I remained in denial that anything seriously untoward was happening, as did my always-capable, always-coping mum. I travelled up from London to see Ella in Glasgow every month or so, sometimes with my family, but it was some time in her eightieth year that I visited her for a weekend alone, also planning to go out one night with friends. Something had changed in her. I told Mum I was having a bath, and went off with a towel. 'Where on earth have you been?' she asked, surprised, as I reappeared damp-haired ten minutes later in her tiny flat. Later, she asked if I was going to have a bath before I went out. I told her no, and explained I was leaving soon to take a present to Maggie, a friend who had just had a baby. My mum remembered Maggie and we chatted about her as we had a cup of tea. Five minutes later Ella began again: 'Who're you here to see?' she asked. 'Maggie. She's had a baby,' I said. 'Oh, that's lovely,' she said. 'Are you having a bath before you go out?'

I wanted to scream and felt completely helpless, watching Ella enter this Möbius strip of purgatory alone. I barely remember the rest of that evening myself, but I know I went out with my girlfriends to a bar on Great Western Road and told them I thought my mum had Alzheimer's. I got so drunk I couldn't cope with the bus, and cried all the way back to her flat in the back of a black taxi. Ella was asleep, but got up early the next morning and looked in on me in the spare bedroom. 'Kate!' she said surprised and pleased. 'I didn't know you were here. When did you arrive from London?'

As the poet Lavinia Greenlaw writes of her father's dementia in *The Sea is an Edge and an Ending*:

The act of forgetting used to take time.
Now it accompanies him through each day
And the world folds itself up behind his every step.[20]

The world had started folding up behind Ella's every step, and there was nothing I could do about it, except get it officially diagnosed.

But I can find out what my generation, and my daughter's, should do, because having a mother with Alzheimer's – not a father – puts you in the higher risk category, though I haven't taken the grim test for the APOE4 gene (which shows increased *risk* of Alzheimer's, not a slam-dunk diagnosis) because I already know the disease runs big-time in my family. So I mostly eat a protective, Mediterranean diet; I stopped drinking alcohol; I run with my dog or a friendly human every day; I have a sloppy relationship with yoga and meditation; I take lots of omega-3 fish oil. Frankly, there's not much else I can do to affect my lifestyle risks of Alzheimer's, except continuing to take estrogen – and testosterone, which puts my brain on fast-forward every morning.

Luckily, I started HRT at 52, a few months after my periods stopped. This is where we come to the interesting 'critical window' hypothesis on the Alzheimer's–estrogen front. In her book, Mosconi notes that: 'Evaluations of the combined statistics of eighteen studies have shown that, among younger 50–59-year-old women, those who took hormones had a 30 to 44 per cent reduced risk of Alzheimer's as compared with those who did not take hormones.'[21] A small 2014 Stanford University study that carried out brain scans of 54 women with a family history of Alzheimer's showed that those using transdermal estrogen had no cognitive decline, while for those using oral estrogen and synthetic progestins the decline was accelerated.[22]

But there's real hope in the findings from the larger Kronos Early Estrogen Prevention Study (KEEPS) in America. Dr Kejal Kantarci, Associate Director at the Mayo Clinic Alzheimer's Disease Research Center, has studied the effects of oral versus transdermal estrogen on 688 menopausal women's brains over seven years.[23] According to Kantarci, 'Participants who took estradiol [estrogen] via skin patches maintained brain volume in the dorsolateral prefrontal cortex, an area of the brain that assists with memory, thinking, planning and reasoning.' And here's the clincher: 'Women who maintained volume in this area of the brain were also more likely to have a lower amount of the amyloid plaque deposits that are related to Alzheimer's disease. This suggests that estradiol therapy may have long-term effects on the brain.'

In another arm of the KEEPS study, Dr Juliana Kling, also at the Mayo Clinic, studied the brain scans of seventy-eight menopausal women and concluded that 'starting HRT in early menopause may reduce risk of dementia and Alzheimer's.'[24] Half the women were given oral or transdermal estrogen with micronised progesterone for two years, and the rest were given a placebo pill. For the women taking estrogen, the hormone had a protective effect: they had fewer white-matter hyperintensities – lesions on the brain indicating cognitive impairment. This messed-up white myelin appears as increased brightness on an MRI brain scan. Kling explains: 'Myelin gives white matter its colour – it helps you think fast, walk straight, and keeps you from falling. When myelin breaks down, the signals can't get through.' Estrogen and perhaps testosterone keep the lines of communication open.

Estrogen not only protects white matter in the brain, but also grey matter in the cerebral cortex, the area essential for attention, memory and learning. Dr Michael Craig, who specialises in female mental health, psychiatry and neuroscience at the Maudsley Hospital in London, started investigating this over ten years ago. In a small study of 61 women, those who used estrogen in the 'critical window' just after menopause maintained their grey matter, while non-users did not.[25] 'I'd like to do a bigger study,' said Craig. 'But since the WHI, it's been really hard to get funded for research involving HRT. It's exasperating.'

Those were all small, hopeful studies, but in May 2021 I actually jumped for joy, and immediately called two friends whose mothers have Alzheimer's disease, as news broke of Dr Brinton's latest research with her fellow scientists at Arizona University.[26] They had studied the health insurance records of almost 400,000 women and discovered that those who had used or were using HRT were 58 per cent less likely to develop Alzheimer's and other neurodegenerative diseases. In fact, those who stayed on HRT longest had the best outcomes: women who took it for six years or more were 79 per cent less likely to develop Alzheimer's and 77 per cent less likely to develop other neurodegenerative diseases like Parkinson's, dementia and multiple sclerosis – a hugely encouraging effect. Brinton explained when the news was released: 'The key is that hormone therapy is not a treatment, but it's keeping the brain and this whole system functioning, leading to prevention. It's not reversing disease; it's preventing disease by keeping the brain healthy.'

The research team was able to see which hormone prescription each woman in the study had used, and the results showed that using body-identical estrogen and progesterone resulted in greater risk reduction than synthetic oral combined hormones. All HRT seemed to help, however. 'Oral hormone therapies resulted in a reduced risk for combined neurodegenerative diseases, while hormone therapies administered through the skin reduced the risk of developing dementia,' the study found. The greatest risk reduction was for patients who are 65 and older.

The Arizona University study is a game-changer, but it still raises all sorts of questions. In particular, to what extent does the timing of hormone use matter? For late adopters, the 'slow drip' theory – starting estrogen in small doses to open up the estrogen receptors gently – may help. After all, if estrogen supplementation over 60 can help with vaginal atrophy, why not brain atrophy too? But perhaps women's brains need protection earlier than 60 in that 'critical window' around the perimenopause and early menopause.

In Britain, there's a growing the-earlier-the-better HRT movement, as women in the perimenopause spot the warning signals of brain fog and memory loss. Dr Shahzadi Harper, a menopause specialist in London, told me that she started taking HRT in her late forties, before menopause, after her mother was diagnosed with Alzheimer's. 'My mum was super-brilliant at arithmetic, had eight children, but at 55 she started getting panic attacks and wouldn't let us shut the bathroom door, she was so anxious. She had sleep apnoea and her memory rapidly got worse.' Her family realised she had Alzheimer's. 'We're Pakistani, so she was already living with my sister and her family, and the rest of us take turns to stay Friday and Saturday and spend the night,' said Harper. After her mother was diagnosed, Harper was on the alert for changes in her own memory. 'I was so scared I was going to develop it too, so three months into feeling perimenopausal I took HRT – I had a good GP, who understood – and I've stayed on it. It has been transformational. If I want to be a doctor, I need my mind to work.'

Different communities have different rates of dementia, and different ways of coping with the illness. Compared with white women, the incidence of dementia diagnosis in the UK is 18 per cent lower among Asian women and 25 per cent higher among Black women, but because there's been no proper study, no one knows whether some cases go under-diagnosed.[27] Allostatic stress, as well as the stress of 'racial weathering', particularly affects some communities. Chronic stress keeps cortisol high, which can lead to premature ageing and onset of Alzheimer's. Once again, there has been very little research into this, or the fact that Black women are less likely to use HRT.[28] Most patients in Alzheimer's studies are white, although efforts are now being made to redress this bias in the scientific community.

Exactly how estrogen positively affects the chances of developing Alzheimer's is not yet clear – is it due to helping with sleep and general health as well as the direct effect on the brain? What's the cumulative effect of the hormones estrogen, progesterone and testosterone on the female brain? Studies have shown that low testosterone levels are associated with the risk of Alzheimer's in elderly men,[29] but we have no data on women. And why are we still asking these questions in 2021, when it has been clear for years that Alzheimer's has very different trajectories in the male and female brain?

Do outdated fears of HRT stop Alzheimer's campaigners from seeing the bigger picture? At the time of writing, the Alzheimer's Society UK charity website had a completely misleading article on hormone replacement therapy that suggested it increased certain types of cancer, heart disease and stroke, again throwing all the different kinds of HRT into one reject basket.[30] Meanwhile, on the Alzheimer's Research UK website, there were two conflicting stories about HRT and

Alzheimer's[31] and the latest science discussed above is missing. When I asked whether there was any forthcoming research about Alzheimer's and estrogen, I received this reply from Dr Rosa Sancho, Head of Research at Alzheimer's Research UK: 'Alzheimer's disease is caused by a complex mix of age, genetics and lifestyle factors – some of which are in our control to change and others aren't. The best current evidence suggests that not smoking, only drinking within the recommended limits, staying mentally and physically active, eating a balanced diet, and keeping blood pressure and cholesterol levels in check can all help to keep our brains healthy . . . Alzheimer's Research UK is currently funding research at the University of Cambridge to further explore why women may have a greater risk of dementia than men, giving greater clarity on a complex area of human biology, which has seen mixed results in previous studies.'

It's all quite vague, and if you've already made the lifestyle changes that Dr Sancho suggests, then where do you go except in the direction of supplementing with estrogen, which has been found to be protective for general health anyway? I don't want to wait around for 20 years for a research paper if I'm entering the early phase of Alzheimer's. I want to do the best I can for my brain right now, based on the evidence available. With that in mind, I talked to Dr Lynne Hughes, who has worked in global neurological research for 30 years, most recently at the healthcare and technology company IQVIA, and has overseen many Alzheimer's clinical trials. She explained: 'Alzheimer's trials take longer to complete, are slower to enrol patients, and are more expensive than other research. The global spend of Alzheimer's research is probably

£3 billion a year, and we have a 99.8 per cent drugs failure rate.' The fact that hormones are not patentable, unlike most drugs, also means major pharmaceutical companies are not interested in investing in expensive trials.

Obviously, estrogen is only part of the picture of what's eating the Alzheimer's brain, and there must be other solutions. In 2020 Bill Gates donated $50 million to Alzheimer's Research UK to help create a mobile app or wearable device that can detect different diseases that cause dementia sooner than we do today, by tracking sleep patterns, gait and eye movements. In his blog, Gates, whose father died of Alzheimer's in 2020, compares the fight against the disease to working on a jigsaw puzzle with his whole family. 'Your goal is to see the whole picture, so that you can understand the disease well enough to better diagnose and treat it. But in order to see the complete picture, you need to figure out how all of the pieces fit together.'[32] Estrogen and testosterone may well be missing pieces of the jigsaw.

Of course, research into male dementia is also essential, but in the meantime the prevailing data indicates that although hormone replacement therapy cannot stop Alzheimer's disease once it has started, it may have the potential to lower the risk of women developing Alzheimer's in the first place if given early enough. HRT is a lifeboat and I'm happy to try it.

Over 40 million people have dementia or Alzheimer's globally, and that means millions more are struggling to care for family members, often giving up their jobs to stay home. As I and many other children of Alzheimer's know, every case of dementia is a shared one. Family, friends or lovers wait helplessly in the wings as communication ebbs away, lost lines no longer respond to prompting, and the curtain falls. Eventually, my mum was looked after almost full-time by carers, one of whom, Helen McArdle, was heroic in her devotion, kindness and ability to bring fun and home-made soup into my mother's life. But while I was away on a week's holiday with my children during a hot August in 2014, the secondary, covering carers from an agency failed to turn up for two days running, and my mother got ill and dehydrated. Ella ended up, upset and muddled, with a urinary tract infection, and in a bed in the Western Infirmary in Glasgow. That day just happened to be what NHS staff dub 'Black Wednesday', when junior doctors all start work in hospitals. This is probably why I found a stranger's drug prescriptions on the clipboard fixed to the end of my mother's bed.

After that was sorted, and it was established Ella had Alzheimer's, a young doctor said: 'Do you want to sign a DNR, then?' I didn't even know what that stood for. *Do Not Resuscitate.* No, I said, but to be honest I had no idea what my mother wanted and had never discussed it with her when she was in good mental health. She was refusing to eat or get out of bed and the nurses had no time to help, so her carer and I went in to feed her every meal for two weeks, a peculiar time when she often thought I was her mother. She never went back to her flat, but left the hospital in a wheelchair for a nursing home, which was staffed by some wonderful, caring, poorly paid women. Ella died in her chair aged 89, after enjoying lunch and a concert.

Is it wrong to use my mother's private life in this public place and to talk about her in her infirmity rather than about how she was so tough, resourceful and intelligent in her earlier years? She never went to university as she had to look after her own mother, who had multiple sclerosis, but became a travelling fur-coat buyer for Great Universal Stores (when that was still a legitimate occupation). Ella was ordering fox furs on the phone when she went into labour with me, and she remained a working mother. She was of that war-child generation that just got on with it: being a carer, a worker and a parent simultaneously, without complaint. Like Margaret Thatcher or the novelist Iris Murdoch, my mother was so much more than her Alzheimer's disease. On the other hand, I don't want anyone else to be a patient or a daughter of Alzheimer's, so if this helps focus attention on the research that still needs to be done, then I'm glad we talked about Ella.

12

THE ANDROPAUSE, MENOPAUSE AND RELATIONSHIPS

Romantic partnerships

'It's not about staying in love with the same person, but falling in love with who that person becomes as they age.'

Helen Juffs, a complementary therapist in her fifties who has been with her partner for 31 years, delivered that piece of menopausal wisdom to me, and I immediately wished she'd been there to tell me that in my forties. For those of us in long relationships, staggering drunkenly into the final years of full-time parenting, there often has to be intentional renewal. Sometimes it's a brutal pruning of the old and a budding of the new, or sometimes it entails breaking away. For some of us, it's less a midlife crisis and more a midlife unravelling. When people talk about 'empty-nest syndrome', there's certainly a moment of grief and joy as offspring spring off, but shouldn't parents consider themselves fledglings too? What will fill the silence and space? Freedom? Boredom? Whoredom? Stardom? Or is it just a chance to take a quiet inventory of your body, of your hormones, and of your frazzled mind, and look after them at last? Because you are not the woman you were in your twenties, and your partner is a very different person too, with his, her or their own middle-aged vulnerabilities. Long-hidden trauma sometimes surfaces. You both have a lot of baggage, and it's unlikely that either of you are professional baggage handlers. That's probably what therapists are for.

Your partner may be in the maelstrom of a midlife crisis too. You are both hitting a half-century, and facing in the direction of death rather than birth, wondering what on earth you're supposed to do. Sometimes you can ride this out together, using the transition as a catalyst for renewal, mutual support and adventure. But many women need to venture out alone for a time at this point, seeking out an alternative reality, a fresh version of themselves, and it's more subtle than the clichés of a lover, a racing bike, a pottery course or a bucket of retinol. Your steady job becomes precarious or boring. Your parents die. You are a very grown-up orphan, and no one is judging you any more. Life teeters on the edge of change.

The menopause can be an engine of extraordinary change, and it can also be a gentle, unspoken slide into compromise in relationships. Actress and presenter Nadia Sawalha – who is also a supporter of The Menopause Charity – made two searingly honest, often funny podcast episodes about the affect her hormonal crash had on her relationship with her husband, television producer Mark Adderley, in the couple's series *How to Stay Married (So Far).*[1] In the two episodes, they discuss the eight-year struggle of living with the menopause in the corner of the room. 'On the marriage side of it, I feel really sorry for both of us, because nobody knew what the hell was going on,' says Sawalha. 'The anxiety was just awful. It was insidious . . . when your hormones go, something shifts in you so much you feel like you're standing on sand.' Sawalha found that her desire just evaporated, much as she loved her husband. 'I couldn't even remember what being a sexual person was like.' Adderley tried to be understanding: 'I dialled that side of myself down a lot,' he said.

The two were in a good relationship, but the strains showed. While she maintained a front for her audience on television, things were very different at home. 'It had just become the norm from three o'clock that I couldn't do anything,' Sawalha says. She was often angry, defensive and irritable, which Adderley found hard. Around menopause, says Sawalha, 'Men are on pause, like they're preserved in aspic. They don't want to do wrong, but they don't know how *not* to do wrong.' She advises men to really 'hug and cuddle your partner with no expectation it will lead to anything else'. Some couples find new depths of connection, or ride this out and move into a new, more platonic phase, while others reach out for medical help or counselling. I wonder how many couples' therapists truly factor hormones into the game. Since the Channel 4 menopause documentary went out and The Menopause Charity offered the free Confidence in the Menopause course to doctors, I've had lots of psychotherapists contacting me asking, *Is there a menopause course for us too?* Not yet. Psychoanalytic psychotherapist Jane Haberlin told me: 'Paradigm shifts are needed. People are pathologising menopause as a mental health issue, when it's about what's happening to the endocrine system. We need to acknowledge that in our work.'

What's interesting about Sawalha and Adderley's relationship is they have seen it from both sides of the homonal divide. After eight years, Sawalha reluctantly decided to try hormone replacement therapy – 'after ten years of looking down my nose at other women' – and she started to feel better, the way she had felt even before having children, and realised that her hormones were to blame. She speaks regretfully to her husband: 'You have been collateral damage in this to a large degree.' But Adderley seems to have cheered up as the podcast ends. 'I have noticed a huge difference in your energy,' he says to Sawalha. 'I've been waiting, babe . . . Shall we go upstairs?'

It is tricky enough for cis couples, but I wondered what happened to some trans men or non-binary people when the menopause unexpectedly erupted, and how relationships would weather that. Even discussing the situation is triggering for many people, but there are websites like queermenopause.com that are leading the conversation for those who want to know more. Long-term use of testosterone may help keep symptoms at bay, but not all trans men use testosterone, and if menopause symptoms do crop up, either after a full hysterectomy or in midlife, it's particularly upsetting. Dr Juliana Kling, who studies menopause and transgender issues at the Mayo Clinic in Minnesota, says: 'There's a lack of data on menopausal transgender patients. We have to extrapolate from menopausal research on female bodies, but what happens to a trans male on high doses of hormones?'

One report in the *Journal of the Endocrine Society* from 2019 tells the story of a 35-year-old plumber, living with his wife and son in Chicago, who had a hysterectomy and his ovaries successfully removed.[2] He was already on testosterone, but following the surgical menopause, he started having hot flushes every hour, and sometimes at night – 'which were very distressing' said the report, 'physically and psychologically'. His doctors upped the testosterone dose, but that just gave him acne and the hot flushes stayed. The doctors considered adding a tiny dose of estradiol (estrogen) to his testosterone – estrogen is a normal male hormone too. 'In our patient, the addition of estradiol presented a particularly unique challenge, because treatment with his gonadal/genetic sex hormone appears to contradict the goal of providing gender-affirming hormone therapy.' But a small dose of estrogen eliminated his hot flushes and 'also resulted in levels of estrogen within the normal range for males, his affirmed sex.' In other words, phew! A year later, the plumber's masculinisation was not affected, his hot flushes were gone and he was once again enjoying being a father and husband.

Most men are attuned to premenstrual tension in their partners and know when to take care or take cover, but the perimenopause and menopause often remain unpredictable mysteries. In a lesbian relationship, there may be double the mood swings, but there's also double empathy. Helen Juffs pointed out that, as two women, lesbian couples always live alongside fluctuating hormones. 'As women together, you find that once a month your mind, your emotions and your hormones can go totally topsy-turvy, and you both have to handle that – and have a good laugh. It's almost like a bank: you pay in the emotions in the good times, and then remember all those moments when you need to be supportive.' Juffs had a much more difficult menopause than her partner, suffering a mixed bag of symptoms from mood swings to genito-urinary problems, until she calmed them with HRT, including vaginal estrogen. 'I was constantly forgetting something, and that can be very annoying. I honestly thought I was getting early-onset dementia.' Fortunately, her partner was very supportive about the forgetfulness. 'To be honest, my relationship with my colleagues at work suffered much more than at home. At one point I had to go into the bathroom to punch the wall to avoid punching a colleague.' She thinks it must be more stressful when two women have a big difference in age and menopauses that are completely out of sync. But at least there's no embarrassment about talking openly. 'My other relationship advice,' said Juffs, laughing, 'is to get a dog.'

Friendships

The menopause and midlife malaise do not drop a bomb merely into sexual relationships; The Change can also alter friendships – for the better, and for the worse. This came as a great surprise to me, not just as someone who got divorced and found, as many do, that many friends feel forced to pick one side in the split. For your friends, the doublethink of talking to both of you is too hard to contemplate, particularly at the early, wounded stages. This is a painful realisation. Also, I have a sense that for married couples there's a fear of toxic contamination from those of us who have left a long-term relationship and leapt irresponsibly into the unknown.

But even before divorce, while my best friends remained rock solid, my other friendships began to change. I was aware that, as the conventional demands of parenting teenagers lessened, and the shadows of the school charity quiz night and the Ford Galaxy people-carrier faded, that I had time to get to know new male, female and multi-gendered colleagues in the film world, where I was a critic, and to campaign for equality and diversity on and behind the screen. A world of powerful, feisty and eccentric women opened up to me, and I felt alive again. Above all, I think midlife is a time in our lives when we need sisterhood, and there's no better place for that than the growing menopause movement. Since I started talking about my own experience, other women have just opened up to me. Every long dog walk together is a revelation.

There also comes a shift in power in midlife friendships, when we realise time is short and we're not going to waste it being polite or hanging out with energy vampires. (*What We Do in the Shadows*, a spoof documentary series about modern-day vampires, has a beige-clad character called Colin who sucks all the positive energy out of the room and bores people to death. We all know one of those.) There's a decisiveness to a midlife woman who has come through the corridor of menopause and slammed the door behind her, and one of the fascinating historical examples of that is the American-born writer Gertrude Stein.

I have been looking forward to discussing the twentieth-century comradeship between the writer Ernest Hemingway, celebrated for his spare prose and über-masculinity, and Stein, celebrated for her avant-garde prose, astute art collection and forthright lesbianism. Stein became a mentor to the young Hemingway when he frequented her salon with other writers and artists in Paris, including Picasso, and later a writerly rivalry erupted. In the 1920s, however, Stein's whole attitude to life and art completely altered with the menopause. She perhaps knew more about it than most of her generation, having trained for four years at medical school, and she probably talked about it privately, which was rare in that time. But the person who was really, really obsessed with Stein's menopause was Hemingway, and he gave the word one of its earliest outings in literature and letters: 'It was the year that she had the menopause that she broke with all her old and good friends,' he observed in one of his letters, after he was suddenly hot-flushed out of her circle.[3] Around that time, Stein's lover, Alice B. Toklas (four years younger and in menopausal range/rage too), was persuaded to give her a short-back-and-sides with the kitchen scissors, and Toklas said, 'The haircut marked a turning point in all sorts of things.' Hemingway linked the crop to the onset of menopause and the beginning of Stein's new 'patriotism' about homosexuality.[4] He moaned that it was an 'unambiguous statement of her sexuality' – though you'd think he'd be used to her lesbianism after 20 or so years of friendship. Now she resembled a monk: an 'imperial ruler, a modernist patriarch'.

As Stein's hair shortened and her self-confidence grew, Hemingway was discombobulated, and possibly a tad emasculated: 'Since the menopause she lost all sense of taste. She could no longer tell a good painting from a bad one, a good writer from a bad one – it all went pftt.'[5] He thought Stein's writing had become lazy, but in 1933, at the age of 59, she published *The Autobiography of Alice. B. Toklas*, which was a modernist sensation. Their literary, personal and hormonal feud gave Hemingway plenty of material, while the notoriously fickle Stein just told her maid to say she wasn't in when he called.

As her estrogen fell, and her testosterone perhaps grew dominant, 'Gertrude's ego grew positively monumental in size,' Hemingway noted after the rift.[6] What if your climacteric ego suddenly gets monumental, you're righteously angry and you just don't give a toss for good taste or what anyone else thinks? Isn't that sometimes wonderful? So many women report feeling loud and liberated in menopause, no longer worrying that their sexuality is upfront in every encounter. So many also talk about feeling an irrational, almost out-of-body rage. They are freed from the need to please, as their caring hormones bail out. But while some women come out fighting, like Stein, around a third of women find menopause destroys their confidence and drags them down, leaving friendships and relationships in peril. A British Menopause Society survey in 2017 found around a quarter of women felt more isolated, and less outgoing in social situations, and a third said they were less active and 'they no longer felt like good company'. Stein felt no such qualms, but then her ego had always been huge: 'No, nobody has done anything to develop the English language since Shakespeare, except myself, and Henry James perhaps a little,' she once said.[7] One of her most famous lines is: 'A rose is a rose is a rose is a rose,' and at one point an angry and rejected Hemingway sent her a copy of his *Death in the Afternoon* with the dedication: 'A bitch is a bitch is a bitch is a bitch.'[8] Final score: Menopause one, Men nil.

The Andropause

Hemingway and Stein got what they deserved from each other – as well as plenty of entertaining and useful material to use for their work. But men are tender creatures, too, in midlife, with similar doubts and fears. The delicate yin and yang of an already established heterosexual relationship can come under hormonal attack from both sides. The male midlife crisis is the stuff of thousands of novels, self-help books, plays and dozens of somewhat age-inappropriate relationships in Woody Allen films. In the arts, the emotional fallout for the heterosexual couple is much discussed, but mostly without factoring in the mad multiverse of the menopause. After all, the coming-of-age novel, essay or film is heavily trod territory, but coming-of-menopause – let's call it coming-of-sage – literature or cinema is rare. In the past few years, that has begun to change, with revelatory midlife writing that often lurks between memoir and fiction and upends the male–female dynamic: Viv Albertine, formerly of the punk band The Slits, in *To Throw Away Unopened*; Deborah Levy's *The Cost of Living*; Bernadine Evaristo's *Girl, Woman, Other*; Darcey Steinke's *Flash Count Diary* and Rachel Cusk's *Kudos*. On screen, the mistress of midlife performance is Frances McDormand with her Oscar-winning performance for Chloé Zhao's *Nomadland*, where she becomes a menopausal Jack Kerouac on the road, in *Three Billboards Outside Ebbing, Missouri,* where her rage is incandescent, and in the television series *Olive Kittridge*, where years of marital resentment are transformed into kinetic energy, scrubbing dishes.

I'm just annoyed that most of those books and films

appeared after my own midlife meltdown, but I thoroughly recommend them. Add that to some medical knowledge and you might think you're sorted, but the missing piece of the picture is what happens to male hormones. Does something transform men when they hit their fifties? Is there a 'male menopause' – or andropause?

As we've noted before, while female progesterone and estrogen disappear during menopause, male testosterone merely goes into gentle decline, so there's no short, sharp shock for men. I talked to Dr Jeff Foster, a men's health specialist with a private GP practice in Warwickshire. He deals with testosterone deficiency in men, prostate and testicular health, and erectile dysfunction, but he's also interested in the wider understanding of the andropause. 'In fact it's more an androslide, since on average men lose about one per cent of their testosterone each year,' he said. '"Andropause" is a cultural term for medical hypogonadism – when you don't produce enough hormones. Testosterone peaks in the late twenties – which is why bodybuilders do well at that age – and then it's downhill.' Foster explained that the effects of testosterone deficiency can include the obvious loss or weakening of erections and libido, but also symptoms in men that are similar to the menopause: fatigue, brain fog, weight gain, depression, lack of energy and, rarely, hot flushes. 'Men don't know they have a problem, because they don't know it exists.' Foster said some men begin to question themselves and their own hormonal state when their partners enter menopause and the storm starts brewing. Foster is also the author of *Man Alive: The Health Problems Men Face and How to Fix Them*[9] and said in many ways the menopause and andropause are very similar, and 'more men would find out about themselves and their relationship if they went to the clinic with their partner.'

Globally around 5 per cent of men over 40 are estimated to suffer low testosterone – some 800,000 in the UK. 'It's a forgotten epidemic,' Dr Foster told me. 'Male menopause is no longer something that should be trivialised or ignored. Men shouldn't feel ashamed or embarrassed about seeing their doctor to discuss a loss of focus, drive, energy, or desire in their life.' A few men experience testosterone deficiency very young, and others need a top up only in later years. Dr Foster said: 'One of my patients was a man in his seventies diagnosed with dementia, but he actually had testosterone deficiency. Brain fog. It wasn't that he couldn't remember things, it was the slowness of recall.' The septuagenarian sharpened up on testosterone. 'I also get a lot of blokes in their fifties who feel they are not as sharp and haven't got that drive any more.'

Unlike women, who know their hormones have bailed when the hot flushes pile on, men need a blood test to learn their testosterone levels, which is usually done in the morning when they're at their highest. Dr Foster advises that if a man has a testosterone level below 12nmol/l (nanomoles per litre), it's probably time for action – although in some areas of the country testosterone supplements only kick in when levels are as low as 7nmol/l. 'Testosterone for men costs about £15 to £45 a month, so the NHS is careful about handing it out,' he says. The NHS only gives out testosterone when levels are extremely low, but the optimal range according to the British Society of Sexual Medicine is higher: therapy is required below 12nmol/l and the recommendation is to aim for a higher target level of 15–30nmol/l in the patient.[10] But is it really a saving for the NHS, leaving lowish testosterone untreated, when after six months benefits begin to show in bone density, muscle mass and cardiovascular health? Just as women get a muffin top in midlife, men sometimes get moobs (man boobs) and beer bellies, as being overweight increases estrogen and lowers testosterone, creating a downward spiral. For some older men, or those with early deficiency, the needs are clear. This is not about dodgy internet testosterone supplements and Instagrammed muscled chests, a cosmetic addition to perfectly healthy levels of hormones. 'What we do is replace what's missing,' says Dr Foster. And keep relationships alive.

The soap-opera cliché of middle-aged men quietly turning to over-the-counter Viagra-type drugs is also true – sales are rising in tandem with penises. Paul Anderson, a consultant urological surgeon in the West Midlands who specialises in genito-urethral reconstruction, has seen everything in this area. Men would rather make a quick purchase than go to the GP's surgery and open up. Pharmacists do consult before purchases, but, says Anderson, 'there's no doctor's consultation with over-the-counter Viagra, and erectile dysfunction is often a signal that there's something else seriously wrong, and it's hidden for years.' That can include low testosterone, diabetes, high blood pressure and cardiovascular disease. In fact, Anderson says that fortunately the 24-hour erectile dysfunction drug tadalafil actually helps lower high blood pressure and reduces mortality rates.[11] In his work, Anderson often sees men in their early fifties: 'They're stressed by the quality of their erection. We can usually help with that, but I've also started asking them about their female partners and whether they have a problem with a dry vagina in perimenopause or menopause. Often the answer's "yes". I give them samples of lubricants and mention topical HRT.' The result is often the return of a successful sex life, on both sides.

Men should know, however, that if they are diagnosed on the NHS with erectile dysfunction, in most areas they will get only eight free pills per month. Twice a week is considered enough healthy British sex, and if you both want more than that, you have to pay over the counter. My friend David, who uses sildenafil (generic Viagra), helpfully points out that this equates to roughly £5 per erection, which could add up to an extra bill of £1,380 a year, were you to engage in nightly activity. I politely refrained from asking him what his top-up costs were, but he was forthcoming anyway: 'It's ball-breakingly expensive.'

Endings and beginnings

It will not surprise you to learn that the peak age for divorce for heterosexual couples is between the ages of 45 and 49, in weird hormonal sync with the perimenopause, and that during that time 62 per cent of divorces are instigated by women.[12] Yes, there are affairs, and children growing up, and the fact we live so long our marriages have to last for half a century. But there is also the kamikaze, *Thelma and Louise* moment that takes a hormonal midlife woman by complete surprise. When I left my marriage, I didn't just regret the hurt I caused to everyone, but the fact that, at the time, I was unable to properly explain to myself or anyone else what had happened. There's an Instagram cartoon truism to cover that: 'Behind every menopausal woman stands a man who has absolutely no idea what he did wrong.' I had little physical baggage at first – my life fitted into ten bin bags and a suitcase in the back of the car; I was glad to escape possessions. I had no idea of the weight of the mental baggage, though, possibly because I was lying beneath it, stoned on some weird perimenopausal trip. There are millions of partners out there filled with goodwill, trying incredibly hard to provide support to a woman who is about to boil over. The lack of honest communication and the 'Keep Calm and Carry On' attitude leaves many women multitasking into oblivion and their partners mystified. You would think doctors might know better, but a male GP once phoned into BBC Radio 4's *Woman's Hour* and said: 'If I had known more about my wife's menopause symptoms, we would still be married.'[13] Same-sex marriage only started in 2014, so those divorce statistics are low, though 72 per of those are between women. But when I look around my world, five apparently-stable heterosexual couples I know broke up in their late forties and early fifties, as did one lesbian couple, all of whom had children in their late teens.

For a younger generation, wild variety and fluidity in sexual relationships is a given. But for those in midlife, raised in more conventional times, a sudden change of heart can be startling. When I was a columnist on the *Times Magazine*, I worked alongside Ginny Dougary, a brilliant and devastating interviewer, who lived with her husband and two sons. Cut to 2021, when I was on Hastings promenade filming for the menopause documentary, with a giant red 'Keep Calm and Carry On' poster featuring a hotlist of symptoms, when Dougary turned up with her wife, MJ Paranzino. 'I'd never had any feelings for women in the past, but when MJ and I kissed, it was as though I were catapulted from one world to another,' said Dougary when I called her later. Paranzino and Dougary are co-founders of the charity Liberty Choir, which create choirs in prisons from prisoners and community volunteers.[14] They met when Dougary was still married, after 20 years with her husband, and working on a book in Provincetown, Massachusetts. 'Volcanic changes come in very long marriages,' said Dougary. In her late forties, a series of life events contributed to the eruption: 'My mother died and I was sucked into the undertow,' she explained, and at the same time Dougary discovered she had hypothyroidism, the symptoms of which can mimic the perimenopause, and was only diagnosed after she went in to the doctor's complaining of heavy periods. She also fell in love with Paranzino: 'I suppose it's late-onset lesbianism. That's LOL.'

The relationship was heady and passionate, intellectually and physically, and a few years later Dougary and Paranzino – who are now in their mid-sixties – found themselves 'menopausing together'. Dougary explained: 'There was definitely a before and after. There was a sudden change in bed in terms of intense body heat. To begin with we could cuddle up and spoon, and now that's quite different, because one of us will suddenly toss all the bedclothes off. We're against separate duvets for aesthetic reasons.' I asked if they had very different experiences of the transition. Dougary was on the phone to me and shouted over to Paranzino in the kitchen: 'You weren't going round with a fan, like me, everywhere you went, were you?' However, Paranzino, who is forthright and funny (and can handle large groups of singing prisoners) was unabashed about her symptoms. Dougary recalled: 'If she was standing in front of the prison choir, she'd just say, "Oh my god, I'm having a hot flush. Can you tell?"' After living together for a few years, the couple got married in 2018. The bride wore a cream silk coat and dress, and the other bride a black tuxedo. 'I love being able to say exactly what I think and do what I want. I feel emboldened,' said Dougary.

But the midlife break-up is not merely of two people, but of a huge organism, often with children at its centre, as well as lifelong friends and family who feel the pain and anxiety alongside you. 'There is, after all, a reason why people battle on being unhappy and unsatisfied in a marriage for the rest of their lives rather than risk change,' said Dougary. There is also the simple horror of waking up alone, well-organised and utterly silent in a rented flat, when you're used to a cheerful home with a cacophony of lost chargers, unfed dogs, last night's empty wine bottles, arguments about the news, rushed plans for the evening, demands for a fiver and cereal packets *put back in the cupboard empty.*

Because of the comic bad timing of menopause, many women find themselves alone just when they are at their most vulnerable. It's hard being a three- or four-day-a-week parent; it feels, at first, like an amputation. Being suddenly single in midlife means you have to make your social life happen rather than letting it wash around you in couply comfort, but it is also a moment where you find out which of your friends have got your back, and as you recover, you can give back to them. High on hormones, I said yes to everything, went to places I'd normally body-swerve, and had a wonderful time. I made fearless and ill-advised decisions to entertain, culminating in a huge Women and Hollywood party to support female film-makers at home, for which my friend Portia made a pie with 'Mash the Patriarchy' written into the potato topping. I then cooked a Burns supper for 50 people by myself (haggis, neeps and tatties are remarkably simple and cheap).

After that, I took the final leap and had a go at online dating, three rocky years after my marriage had ended. I am a very nosey person, and online dating turned out to be absolutely fascinating: somewhere between anthropology, zoology and psychology, with added unpredictable drama. The midlife dating industry offers huge choice – there is even myLovelyParent, in which grown children post entries recommending their mum or dad. (I didn't do that. I wasn't sure if I'd get a good reference.) I chose a website that no longer exists, Guardian Soulmates, which involved detailed, pretentious biographies and hobbies, a whole album of sporty or arty-farty pictures, and loads of longwinded messaging before anyone ever considered proposing a cup of mint tea. Perfect for me. I was terrified of something like Tinder or Bumble, which involves instant swiping, since I am directionally challenged and often don't know my left from my right. I always have the wrong leg up in yoga.

I read an article about Holly Martyn, a newly divorced mother who took a courageous decision to keep dating, whatever happened, for a year and wrote *Would It Kill You to Put on Some Lipstick?: 1 Year and 100 Dates*. I vowed not to be cowed by age, rejection or lunatics, but to plough on (though I was mildly creeped out by the many profiles of my contemporary 50-something men that indicated they would only date women ten or more years younger than them. Just say no to the menopause, lads!). But there were some fantastic men out there, mostly battered from divorce and full of hard-earned wisdom, just like the women. I looked upon each so-called date with a stranger – mostly a dog-walk in the park, occasionally a drink – less as a potential romance and more a way to winkle out a life story. Safer that way. I made friends. I met a wreck diver, a Scottish Nationalist, a documentary maker, a psychotherapist and an academic with an interest in Masonic aprons, who made the cardinal error of failing to ask my dog's name on our walk.

Then a message appeared in the dating inbox from a friend I'd first met aged 17, in my law class at Glasgow University. I hadn't seen him since we graduated, over three decades earlier. We went out for dinner and talked so much we didn't eat the food. A few weeks later, we took my somewhat useless dog, Skye, for a walk in Highgate Woods and after about ten minutes she shot after a squirrel and disappeared into the undergrowth. For the duration of the ensuing nerve-wracking and embarrassing search, my new-old friend remained calm and encouraging. After half an hour, I got a call saying there was a lost dog at the gate by the pub. Instinctively, she had headed for a drink. We picked Skye up and went for coffee. We're still together.

13

FEMINISM AND THE FUTURE

When the menopause first rolled in, it weighed upon me like a heavy tyre dumped in my lap. Then, after I turned to others for help, the tyre fell to the ground and I began slowly rolling it uphill. Soon I realised there were women everywhere around me pushing tyres: activists, doctors, writers, patients, academics and Instagrammers, the menopause movement that helped make this book, the documentary, and The Menopause Charity. Together at the top, we released hundreds of tyres and they rolled downhill, faster and faster, exploding myths in their path, bouncing with delightful unpredictability into the future.

One by one, those tyres will smash the frame built by the patriarchy around this conversation centuries ago – with witch-hunts, purgatives and leeching, and asylums for hysterics and hags. Then the menopause will find its rightful cultural and medical space in the world. No longer will we fade away and lose our marbles, if we can help it. The confluence of ageism and sexism that made us 'invisible and unfuckable', as director Jane Campion once said, will eventually be vanquished. We will party, protest, joyfully fuck, and tell the world that menopause is a human rights issue. That women over 50 are no longer dispensable and disposable, but a key part of the workforce and lifeforce. 'It has always been about keeping women invisible and not normalising the conversation around menopause as we get older. That absolutely fuels the age-centric, youth-centric conversation,' says Omisade Burney-Scott in her US podcast *The Black Girl's Guide to Surviving the Menopause.*[1] 'Your usefulness and value in this country is diminished, and you and I know that is absolutely not true.' Her mission – and it's great and sometimes wacky listening – is 'normalising menopause and aging by centring the stories of Black women, femmes and non-binary people. It's our time!'

Demystifying the menopause is half the battle, but we must also challenge the medical canon and get the facts out there – that menopause is a long-term hormonal deficiency that can be easily fixed. We can make menopause symptoms history for most women, and in the process vastly improve their quality of life and long-term health. Another powerful podcaster (and podcasts are a surprising engine for menopausal change) is the UK's former glossy-magazine editor Lorraine Candy, whose *Postcards from Midlife* podcast with Trish Halpin often mainlines menopause in extraordinary women's life stories. The more Candy investigates and hears of women being refused help, the more she finds the institutional sexism in medicine and society unconscionable. One morning she just got on the phone to me and stormed: 'Why don't we deserve the best? Not giving us replacement hormones is like kidnapping us and keeping us in an emotional cellar. Why does this culture want to stop a lot of women over 50 from having sex? We're free of childbearing and -rearing, we're ourselves again, but society has done with us. HRT liberates women.' As

Davina McCall said to me as we plotted the a second documentary focusing on midlife women in the workplace, 'The question we need to ask this time is not *Why should I take HRT?*, but *Are there any reasons at all why I shouldn't?*'

The answer to it all is education, education, education, for women themselves and for doctors – and politicians. One of the trustees of The Menopause Charity is Dr Radhika Vohra, a Surrey GP and menopause specialist, and when we spoke she was partway through giving NHS training in women's health to 90 GPs. 'The menopause programme available is dire,' said Dr Vohra. 'There are a third more doctors' appointments made by women than men, and we're not responding enough to that need, some of which is around menopause.' Vohra works with a large Asian community: 'For older women, the long-term health risks are huge, post-menopause – diabetes, bone health, heart disease . . . The NHS website is very limited and incredibly vague. I have lots of middle-aged women in, talking about "all-over body pain" – if they're eating a plant-rich diet, they don't always present with hot flushes – and they don't know help is available.'

We need more literature in different languages, so that menopause knowledge is not just for the privileged. Even if you don't want medical help, just knowing what is going on with your body can make a difference and allay fears. We don't all have to be pro HRT, but we should all be pro giving women the choice. There isn't a leaflet in any language on the menopause in my doctor's surgery, something which could be easily fixed. Even just a poster of menopause symptoms, like the downloadable Pausitivity posters (in English, Welsh, Urdu, Gaelic, German and Dutch, thus far) that you can print off and take into your surgery for the noticeboard[2] – again, a case of sisters doing it for themselves. Another utterly simple solution would be for GPs to give every woman over 40 a list of menopause symptoms to tick off, and which can open discussion.

However loud the calls for change, the medical establishment moves slowly, and – rightfully – carefully. Sometimes the medical motto 'First, do no harm' weighs heavily against change or seeing the big picture. Many doctors think the safest way to handle the menopause is to ignore it, rather than intervene, and a huge body of evidence linking the old combined HRT to a small risk of breast cancer stands in the way of helping women's long-term health. But senior menopause experts are challenging the orthodoxy and the lack of new research, and just getting on with prescribing the best possible HRT to women, while the system catches up.

Once you see the long-term health picture, everything clicks into place. One in two women get osteoporosis. One in five get Alzheimer's. What if most didn't? The savings would be monumental. I'm not a health economist, but I can do basic arithmetic and the small cost of giving women the best HRT at £120 a year, for estrogen and progesterone, is massively offset by decreased repeat visits to the GP in the short-term and health protection into the future. Two million women in the UK have osteoporosis, and around 350,000 arrive in hospital with fragility fractures every year, costing the NHS around £3 billion.[3] Mental ill-health costs the NHS £94 billion a year, cardiovascular disease £19 billion, diabetes £6 billion and dementia £26 billion. What if we could vastly reduce those bills?

The women's movement also needs to be publicly honest about the devastating consequences of the menopause for many and about its long-term health risks, and to make it clear that empowering women with knowledge and handing them a mini desk-fan may not be quite enough. Baroness Sayeeda Warsi, a peer in the House of Lords, bravely came onto the menopause documentary and talked openly about her brain fog during menopause – and her memory loss on the floor of the upper chamber when she was in the middle of a political speech. She made lifestyle changes to combat her menopause, and on camera as she lifted spectacularly large weights in a gym, she explained her biggest concern: 'How do we have this conversation, which allows women to be supported and understood during this time but without making this a stick with which men can then beat us and say, "Ah, we always said women couldn't be as good as men. We always said they weren't up to the job"? The more we start to raise it in the public sphere, the more we're not hiding this, the more we're not ashamed of this. One of my daughters is a medic and she always says, "If men had menopause, we'd have fixed it by now."'

If men had menopause, the science would be spectacular. Dr Pauline Maki, who has been studying the role of female hormones on the brain for 20 years at the University of Illinois in Chicago, is calling for more Alzheimer's research. 'There is so much paternalism round everything hormonal. I think women need to demand this kind of work,' she says. 'More women need to tell their stories. You don't want to pathologise menopause, generally; it's not a problem for most. But if we fail to recognise that it is a problem for a certain percentage of women, then we do women a tremendous amount of harm.'[4]

Just writing this book, and interviewing pioneering male and female doctors and academics across four continents, has made me realise that the picture of the menopause is lying in jigsaw pieces in scientific silos all over the world, waiting to be joined up. The more we raise consciousness about the menopause, the quicker that jigsaw will be finished. We need to understand more about the menopause experience – medically and otherwise – in other cultures, and to track the inequalities in developing countries. Right now, accurate menopause knowledge and hormone replacement remain unattainable luxuries in some countries, but in the way that some other hormones have become mainstream corrective medicine – insulin for diabetes, and thyroxin for thyroids – so might HRT.

A shout-out here to the woman who discovered how to measure hormones like estrogen and insulin in the blood. I hadn't heard of Dr Rosalyn Yalow, but she has had a profound effect on my life and the lives of billions of others. In 1977 she became the second woman to win a Nobel Prize for medicine – for her radioimmunoassay hormone-detecting technique. In reference to Dr Yalow, the Nobel committee said: 'We are witnessing the birth of a new era of endocrinology.' Yalow, who started out as a nuclear physicist, was first interested in tracking insulin, as her husband had diabetes, but struggled to get a research position as a woman and mother of two, and at first made her laboratory in a janitor's closet in a hospital in the Bronx, New York, where she worked. Like I said, sisters doing it for themselves.

And talking of sisters, we also need to join hands with the younger generation of intersectional feminists, learn from the Period Power generation, and march forward together. As Minna Salami writes in *Sensuous Knowledge: A Black Feminist Approach for Everyone*,[5] 'I did not want to write a protest book, I wanted to write a progress book.' And that's what I want to do here. Now we've protested and now that we understand the science, we need to make progress. 'We must be the last generation of women suffering like this,' says Dr Louise Newson. And if there's one woman in the UK who's made a difference to menopause, it's Dr Newson. The evidence-based knowledge gathered in her constantly updated, non-commercial balancemenopause.com site is far better and more comprehensive than anything the NHS produces, and the site also talks holistically about the menopause, from nutrition to microbiomes to yoga, and what women can do dealing with difficult conditions post cancer. There are over a hundred podcasts on the site, with subjects ranging from endometriosis to relationships. Dr Newson's free Balance Menopause Support app (which has one of the most comprehensive symptoms lists you'll ever enjoy reading) has been downloaded by over a quarter of a million women in over half the countries of the world, so the appetite for knowledge is out there. Over 1 billion women will be menopausal or postmenopausal by 2030 – 12 per cent of the world's population – and the upcoming Generation X will be silent no more. Perhaps it's time for a new wave of feminism, a tsunami of perimenopausal and menopausal women kicking ageism into touch and demanding better information and health outcomes for a billion of their sisters around the world. Time's Up for marginalising the menopause.

Fem-tech and meno-tech will help us move forward, even if ingrained medical sexism is holding us back. Erica Opare, who created Liria Digital Health in Leeds after realising what her mother had gone through in silence after a hysterectomy-induced menopause, expects that meno-tech will be huge. 'Over fifty per cent of the global population is not niche, and menopause has been under the radar until now.' As a Black British woman who previously worked in NHS tech, Opare is aware of 'the Black and ethnic minority barrier to healthcare. The culture for my mum was just to grin and bear it.' She is gathering data, researching what's needed, and hopes to help the NHS make a digital leap forward. 'Knowledge is power, and giving women access to information and a community spirit through an app could make a huge difference.'

Pioneering change also starts on the ground. The brilliant Menopause Café[6] movement basically works like a vast menopausal book group – symptoms and life-changes are discussed over coffee and cake, and it provides a 'respectful, confidential space, open to everyone, regardless of gender or age', says its founder, Rachel Weiss. The website helps you create an event, where there is no prescribed agenda and people swap tables to meet each other in small groups. 'Menopause isn't just about the physical and psychological changes – it's about the philosophical ones too,' Weiss says. Obviously, you could also convene in your own Menopause Pub somewhere, or create a menopause WhatsApp philosophy group, or join the #MakeMenopauseMatter campaign.[7] I'm considering starting a Menopause Roadshow with other menopause warriors and doctors. We need to harness expertise, menopausal rage and humour to change. We need to be inspired by the early work of comedians like Joan Rivers, who left her audience squirming and squealing with such lines as: 'The vagina drops. One morning, I woke up and thought, *Why am I wearing a bunny slipper? And why is it grey?*'

Every day, as @menoscandal, I plunge into a vast Instagram and Twitter community of menopause activists – a window into other worlds. While middle-class white women are fighting for care and attention, and often getting it, many communities do not see themselves reflected in the menopause movement. Hence Dr Nighat Arif's menopause TikToks in Urdu,[8] Michelle McCarthy's resource pack for helping menopausal women with learning disabilities,[9] Tania Glyde's queermenopause.com, Karen Arthur's @menopausewhilstblack Instagram and podcasts and Nina Kuypers' @BLKMenopause on Twitter and Black Women in Menopause Facebook group. Karen Arthur puts the case succinctly and powerfully in one of her posts: 'Racial weathering is the constant wearing-down effect of racism on black people's physical and mental wellbeing. From micro-aggressions to murder. Knowing it, seeing it, feeling it, living it. Every single day. It may explain why many Black women experience menopause up to two years earlier and more severely than our white counterparts . . . I will say this to menopausal and non-menopausal Black women – Up Your Self Care Game.'

Kuypers founded the Facebook group after her own difficult experience. 'The images and experience of menopause in the mainstream media didn't resonate for me,' Kuypers says. 'There were no platforms posing questions about the changes for Black women – my *Fraggle Rock* hair, my polka-dot skin, my different cultural experiences – so I made this safe space where Black women and women of colour could have open discussions. I think of menopause as a holiday where we all have different suitcases and different destinations to land in, psychologically, physically and emotionally.' Her online events quickly filled up. 'I can't find the words to describe so much lovely feedback,' she says. It is clear that social media is key to support and change, especially when the medical establishment and the culture is so set in its crusty ways.

The revolution must happen worldwide, and we should not be unambitious about that, though here in the UK we just need one, intelligent government minister to understand how a few simple, cheap changes could have a profound effect on almost every women's health, long term happiness and economic productivity. We need a health service that offers all women an informed choice, and does not leave behind the marginalised and economically deprived. We need to be offered estrogen, progesterone and testosterone for our long-term health and not just our short-term symptoms, and in the process save the NHS billions. We need to bring government policy on the menopause into the twenty-first century and help all female employees survive and thrive during this transition. And we need to fund women-centric research on a vast scale.

We women also just need to fall back in love with our bodies after menopause and look after them holistically, and to pay equal attention to our souls, left ragged after half a century of multitasking. We need to hold hands and make the great leap forward – from Period Power to Menopause Power.

We need to talk about the menopause. We need to make the menopause about metamorphosis, not misery. We need tell our mad, moving menopause stories to the women and men and children in our lives. We are the links in the menopausal chain of silence that goes back beyond our mothers and grandmothers, and we must break that chain to free ourselves and our daughters. Go out there and tell your story.

ACKNOWLEDGEMENTS

This book would not exist had I not met the extraordinary Dr Louise Newson, my menopause guru in all things scientific, and a tireless campaigner for women excluded from healthcare. Huge gratitude goes to her and the menopause specialists at Newson Health and The Menopause Charity. In particular, I would like to thank Dr Zoe Hodson, Dr Radhika Vohra, and Dr Rebecca Lewis for their expert advice. Every doctor, academic and menopause specialist interviewed here gave generously of their time, especially Dr Nighat Arif, Dr Paula Briggs, Dr Shahzadi Harper, Mr Nick Panay, Professor Philip Sarrel, Professor Michael Baum and Dr Avrum Bluming.

My research was done in tandem with making the documentary, *Sex, Myths and the Menopause*, presented by Davina McCall, and her honesty and dedication kept us all going as we filmed in lockdown. Thanks also to the team at Finestripe Productions in Glasgow, director Linda Sands, executive producer Katie Lander, and Dorothy Byrne, who commissioned the programme at Channel 4 and believed in us from the start.

My agent Sheila Crowley at Curtis Brown was instrumental in creating the tone of this book and supporting me throughout. I'm also delighted to have worked with Fritha Saunders and Kat Ailes, my editors at Simon and Schuster, who provided much-needed scaffolding for the outpouring of words, and wise advice.

The growing menopause movement in the UK has been key to this story, and big thanks go to Carolyn Harris MP, Katie Taylor of The Latte Lounge, Menopause Charity ambassador Liz Earle, Lorraine Candy of *Postcards from Midlife*, Sarah Davies of Talking Menopause, Diane Danzebrink of #MakeMenopauseMatter and Justine Roberts of Mumsnet for their campaigning work.

Every chapter was built on the stories of friends and strangers who became allies in the collaborative telling of our menopausal experience. In particular I'd like to thank Kirsty Lang, Pat Hood, Ann Newson, Louisa Young, Portia Kamons, Deborah Ross, Ginny Dougary, Kate Macfarlane, Vanora Bennett, Karen Mullis, Gill Morgan, Helen Juffs, Clare Longrigg, Rowan Pelling, Stephanie Theobald, Karen Arthur, Sam Evans, Kate Duffy, Hayley Cockman, So Mayer, Lizzie Francke, and Nancy Bond. My final thanks go to my children Molly, Barney and Finn Macintyre for their support, and my partner Cameron Scott, who gave me the space, time and love that made writing possible.

MENOPAUSE SUPPORT RESOURCES

Balance App
Free menopause app with symptom tracker and HRT advice.
balance-app.com

The Daisy Network
Support and networking for young women with early menopause and premature ovarian insufficiency.
www.daisynetwork.org

The Eve Appeal
Gynaecological cancer research charity raising awareness around womb, ovarian, cervical, vulval and vaginal cancer.
www.eveappeal.org.uk

Endometriosis Charity
Support, advice and community for women with endometriosis.
www.endometriosis-uk.org

Henpicked
Advice for working women during the menopause.
henpicked.net

The Latte Lounge
Online platform offering support and information on health and wellbeing for women during midlife.
www.lattelounge.co.uk/menopause

LGBTQIA+ Menopause
Inclusive research site with connections for trans men, non-binary and intersex people, among others.
www.queermenopause.com

Meg's Menopause
Friendly, accessible advice from Brit-pop icon turned menopause campaigner Meg Mathews.
www.megsmenopause.com

Menopause Café
Create your own local menopause support group.
www.menopausecafe.net

The Menopause Charity
Advice and campaigning website, with sections for employers and health professionals.
www.themenopausecharity.org

Menopause in the Workplace
Advice and training for employers and employees.
www.menopauseintheworkplace.co.uk

Menopause Support

Information and support for women and their families. Home of the national #MakeMenopauseMatter campaign.
www.menopausesupport.co.uk

M-powered Women

Support and advice site on menopause and wellbeing.
www.mpoweredwomen.net

My Menopausal Vagina

Advice on genito-urinary symptoms of menopause, dry vagina, and vaginal atrophy (in English and Urdu).
www.mymenopausalvagina.co.uk

Balance Menopause

Evidence-based medical and holistic information and over a hundred podcasts from menopause specialist Dr Louise Newson.
www.balance-menopause.com

NHS NICE guidelines on the menopause

Advice on care GPs should provide. You can take these to your GP as guidance.
www.nice.org.uk/guidance/ng23

Ovacome

Charity supporting women in surgical menopause after the removal of ovaries.
www.ovacome.org.uk

Talking Menopause

Training from consultants, coaches and specialists raising awareness of the menopause at work.

www.talkingmenopause.co.uk

Women's Health Concern

Medical menopause information from the British Menopause Society.

www.womens-health-concern.org

Menopause Instagram accounts:

@menoscandal, @menopausewhilstblack, @drnighatarif, @dianedanzebrink, @prematuremenopause14, @themenocharity, @menopause_doctor, @motheringandthemenopause, @jane_thepelvicfloorbible

FURTHER READING

Baker, Sam, *The Shift: How I Lost and Found Myself After 40 – and You Can Too* (London: Coronet, 2020)

Bluming, Avrum and Tavris, Carol P., *Oestrogen Matters* (London: Piatkus, 2018)

Criado Perez, Caroline, *Invisible Women: Exposing Data Dias in a World Designed for Men* (London: Chatto and Windus, 2019)

D'Souza, Christa, *The Hot Topic: A Life Changing Look at the Change of Life* (London: Short Books, 2016)

Earle, Liz, *The Good Menopause Guide* (London: Orion, 2018)

Harris, Jane (ed.), *M-Boldened: Menopause Conversations* (Cheltenham: Flint Books, 2020)

Hill, Maisie, *Perimenopause Power: Navigating Your Hormones on the Journey to Menopause* (London: Green Tree, 2021)

Lewis, Jane, *Me and My Menopausal Vagina* (Great Britain: PAL Books, 2018)

Mathews, Meg, *The New Hot: Taking on the Menopause with Attitude and Style* (London: Vermillion, 2020)

Mattern, Susan P., *The Slow Moon Climbs: The Science, History and Meaning of the Menopause* (Princeton University Press: Princeton, 2019)

Mosconi, Lisa, *The XX Brain: The Groundbreaking Science Empowering Women to Prevent Dementia* (London: Allen & Unwin, 2020)

Newson, Louise, *Menopause: All You Need to Know in One Concise Manual* (Yeovil: Haynes Publishing, 2019)

Newson, Louise, *Preparing for the Perimenopause and Menopause* (London: Penguin, 2021)
Panay, Nick, Briggs, Paula, Kovacs, Gabor T. (eds), *Managing the Menopause: Second Edition* (Cambridge: Cambridge University Press, 2020)
Sheehy, Gail, *The Silent Passage* (New York: Random House, 1992)
Simpson, Jane, *The Pelvic Floor Bible* (London: Penguin, 2019)
Steinke, Darcey, *Flash Count Diary* (New York: Farrar, Straus & Giroux, 2019)
Theobald, Stephanie, *Sex Drive* (London: Unbound, 2018)

NOTES

CHAPTER 1: THE REVOLUTION STARTS HERE

1 Hunter, M. S., Gentry-Majaraj, A., Ryan, A., et al, 'Prevalence, frequency and problem rating of hot flushes persist in older post-menopausal women: impact of age, body mass index, hysterectomy, hormone therapy use, lifestyle and mood in a cross-sectional cohort study of 10,418 British women aged 54–65', *British Journal of Obstetrics and Gynaecology*, 2012, 119(1): 40–50.

2 Chunn, L, 'Leading psychotherapist Susie Orbach explains why every middle aged woman needs therapy', dailymail.co.uk, November 2016.

3 Mundy, L. 'The secret power of menopause', *The Atlantic*, October 2019.

4 Ibid.

5 Mattern, S., *The Slow Moon Climbs: The Science, History, and Meaning of Menopause* (Princeton University Press, 2019).

6 Nattrass, S., Croft, D. P., Ellis, S., et al., 'Post-reproductive killer whale grandmothers improve the survival of their grandoffspring', *Proceedings of the National Academy of Sciences of the United States of America*, 2019, 115(52): 26669–73.

7 Ratcliffe. J., '"Brokenness and holiness really go together": Darcey Steinke on menopause', Longreads.com, June 2019.

8 Steinke, D., 'Flash Count Diary: Menopause and the Vindication of Natural Life', (Picador, 2019) p.215.

9 Ibid., p.215.

10 Channel 4/Fawcett Society Menopause and the Workplace Survey, 2022, fawcettsociety.org.uk/menopauseandtheworkplace

11 Wolff, J., 'What doctors don't know about menopause', *AARP The Magazine*, August/September 2018.
12 Willi, J., Süss, H., Grub, J. et al., 'Biopsychosocial predictors of depressive symptoms in the perimenopause – findings from the Swiss Perimenopause Study', *Menopause*, 2021, 28(3): 247–54.
13 Bansal, R. and Aggarwal, N., 'Menopausal hot flashes', *Journal of Mid-Life Health, 2019, 10(1): 6–13.*
14 'Estrogen may relieve post-menopausal joint pain, study suggests', Sciencedaily.com, March 2013.
15 Gayatri, D., 'Menopause-Related Cognitive Impairment', *Obstetrics & Gynecology*, 2018, 312(6) 1325–7.
16 Oliver, M., 'Katharina Dalton, 87; First Doctor to Define, Treat PMS', *Los Angeles Times*, September 2004.
17 'What your mother never told you about health with Dr Sharon Malone', *The Michelle Obama Podcast*, August 2020.
18 Brewis, J., Beck, V., Davies, A., et al., 'Menopause transition: effects on women's economic participation', gov.uk, July 2017.
19 Newson, L., 'Menopause and the Workplace', newsonhealth.co.uk
20 Criado Perez, C., *Invisible Women: Exposing Data Bias in a World Designed for Men* (Chatto & Windus, 2019).
21 'Testosterone replacement in menopause', thebms.org.uk.
22 'Are women suffering in silence? New survey puts spotlight on significant impact of menopause despite recent guideline', thebms.org.uk, May 2016.
23 Glyde, T., 'How can therapists and other healthcare practitioners best support and validate their queer menopausal clients?', *Sexual and Relationship Therapy*, February 2021; article abstract available at tandfonline.com.
24 Velez, A., 'Menopause is different for women of color', endocrineweb.com.
25 'How depression and menopause freed Karen Arthur', *Stylelikeyou*, YouTube.com, August 2019.
26 Ellis, R., 'Why *do* so many GPs refuse to give women HRT? Patients are struggling with menopausal symptoms – and expert consensus is that hormone treatment is safe', dailymail.co.uk, June 2018.
27 Moran, C., "Me, drugs and the perimenopause." thetimes.co.uk, July 2020.
28 'Hormone replacement therapy (HRT): Types', nhs.uk.
29 Muir, K., 'Half of us go through it, yet doctors till aren't being taught about the menopause: As women struggle with hot flushes, fuzzy

memory and low mood, a charity founder reveals shameful lack of training given to GPs', dailymail.co.uk, 24 May 2021.

30 nuffieldtrust.org.uk/resource/chart-of-the-week-hormone-replacement-therapy-prescriptions-rise-42-in-one-year

31 'Menopause Support survey reveals shocking disparity in menopause training in medical schools', menopausesupport.co.uk, May 2021.

32 'MNHQ here: results of our survey about the menopause, perimenopause and experiences with GPs', mumsnet.com, February 2020.

33 'Clinical topic guides', rcgp.org.uk

34 Greer, G., *The Change* (Bloomsbury, 2018), p.33.

35 Lorde, A., *A Burst of Light: Essays by Audre Lorde* (Firebrand Books, 1988).

36 'What are your chances of living to 100?' ons.gov.uk, January 2016.

37 Mosconi, L., Rahman, A., Diaz, I., et al., 'Increased Alzheimer's risk during the menopause transition: A 3-year longitudinal brain imaging study', *PLoS ONE*, 2018, 13(12): e0207885.

CHAPTER 2: NOT WAVING BUT DROWNING

1 Smith, S., 'Not Waving but Drowning', 1972, poetryfoundation.org.

2 Sheng, Y., Carpenter, J. S., Elomba, C. D., et al., 'Review of menopausal palpitations measures', *Women's Midlife Health*, 2021, 7(5).

3 Channel 4/Fawcett Society Menopause and the Workplace Survey, 2022, fawcettsociety.org.uk/menopauseandtheworkplace

4 Menopause Test Kit blurb, superdrug.com.

5 Channel 4/Fawcett Society Menopause and the Workplace Survey, 2022, fawcettsociety.org.uk/menopauseandtheworkplace

6 Moran, C., 'Caitlin Moran: Me, drugs and the perimenopause', *The Times*, July 2020.

7 Graville, S., 'Menopause & me: Skye Gyngell', mpoweredwomen.net, April 2019.

8 D'Souza, C., *The Hot Topic* (Short Books, 2016).

9 Channel 4/Fawcett Society Menopause and the Workplace Survey, 2022, fawcettsociety.org.uk/menopauseandtheworkplace

10 Carpenter, S., 'Forgetful? Befuddled? Blame the Pink Fog: You read the same book twice and don't realise. You hunt for your phone as you chat on it. Don't panic, you've just hit a certain age!' dailymail.co.uk, August 2012.

11 'Menopause survey results published!' newsonhealth.co.uk, March 2019.

12 Duncan, P. and Marsh, S., 'Antidepressant use in England soars as pandemic cuts counselling access', *Guardian*, January 2021.
13 'Menopause: Diagnosis and Management', nice.org.uk, December 2019.
14 Wise, J., 'One in 10 women in England takes antidepressants, survey shows', bmj.com, 2014: 349.
15 Brody, D. J. and Qiuping Gu, M. D., 'Antidepressant Use Among Adults: United States, 2015–2018', National Center for Health Statistics, September 2020.
16 Gordon, J. L., Rubinow, D. R., Eisenlohr-Moul, T. A., et al., 'Efficacy of transdermal oestradiol and micronized progesterone in the prevention of depressive symptoms in the menopause transition: a randomized clinical trial', *JAMA Psychiatry*, 2018, 75(2): 149–57.
17 'Menopause: Diagnosis and Management', op. cit.
18 Rosenhek, J., 'Mad with menopause', doctorsreview.com, February 2014.

CHAPTER 3: HORMONES: THE HOLY TRINITY – ESTROGEN, PROGESTERONE AND TESTOSTERONE

1 Kay, C., 'Over 50s market prefers "enhancement" to anti-ageing', *raconteur.net*, September 2015.
2 Thornton, M. J., 'Estrogens and aging skin', *Dermato-Endocrinology*, 2013, 52(1): 264–70.
3 Cui, J., Shen, Y. and Li, R., 'Estrogen synthesis and signaling pathways during ageing: from periphery to brain', *Trends in Molecular Medicine*, 2013, 19(3): 197–209.
4 Bhupathiraju, S. N., Grodstein, F., Rosner, B. A., et al., 'Hormone therapy use and risk of chronic disease in the Nurses' Health Study: a comparative analysis with the Women's Health Initiative', *American Journal of Epidemiology*, 2017, 186(6): 696–708.
5 Botteri, E., Støer, N. C., Sakshaug, S., et al., 'Menopausal hormone therapy and colorectal cancer: a linkage between nationwide registries in Norway', *BMJ Open*, 2017: e017639.
6 Salpeter, S., R., Walsh, J. M. E., Ormiston, T. M., et al., 'Meta-analysis: effect of hormone-replacement therapy on components of the metabolic syndrome in postmenopausal women', *Diabetes, Obesity and Metabolism*, 2006, 8(5): 538–54.

7 Dr Avrum Bluming and Carol Tavris, *Oestrogen Matters* (London, Piatkus, 2018).

8 Zetterberg., M., 'Age-related eye disease and gender', *Maturitas*, 2016, 83: 19–26.

9 Gross s., and Whipple E., Menopause and Multiple Sclerosis, msfocus-magazine.org, 2020.

10 Gold, S. and Voskuhl, R. R., 'Estrogen treatment in multiple sclerosis', *Journal of the Neurological Sciences*, 261(1–2): 99–103.

11 'What women need to know', nof.org.

12 Benedetti, M. G., Furlini, G., Zati, A., et al., 'The effectiveness of physical exercise on bone density in osteoporotic patients', *BioMed Research International*, 2018: 4840531.

13 Cheraghi, Z., Doosti-Irani, A., Almasi-Hashiani, A., et al., 'The effect of alcohol on osteoporosis: a systematic review and meta-analysis', *Drug and Alcohol Dependence*, 2019, 197: 197–202.

14 Naves Diaz, M., O'Neill, T. W. and Silman, A. J., 'The influence of alcohol consumption on the risk of vertebral deformity. European Vertebral Osteoporosis Study Group', *Osteoporosis International*, 1997, 7(1): 65–71.

15 Thomas, P. A., 'Racial and ethnic differences in osteoporosis', *Journal of the ASOS*, 2007, 15: S26–S30.

16 Louisa Young, *You Left Early: A True Story of Love and Alcohol* (The Borough Press, 2018).

17 'Prevention and treatment of osteoporosis in women', thebms.org.uk, 2018.

18 Davis, L. S. 'Why modern medicine keeps overlooking menopause', *New York Times*, April 2021.

19 'Coronavirus (COVID-19) related deaths by ethnic group, England and Wales: 2 March 2020 to 15 May 2020', ons.gov.uk, June 2020.

20 Newson, L., Manyonda, I., Lewis, R., et al., 'Sensitive to infection but strong in defense – female sex and the power of oestradiol in the Covid-19 pandemic', *Frontiers in Global Women's Health*, May 2021.

21 Sudre, C. H., Murray, B., Varsavsky, T., et al., 'Attributes and predictors of long-Covid: analysis of Covid cases and their symptoms collected by the Covid Symptoms Study App', medrxiv.org, October 2020.

22 Dambha-Miller, H., Hinton, W., Joy, M., et al., 'Mortality in Covid-19 amongst women on hormone replacement therapy or combined oral contraception: a cohort study', medrxiv.org, February 2021.

23 Al-kuraishy, H. M., Al-Gareeb, A. I., Faidah, H., et al., 'The looming

effect of estrogen in Covid-19: a rocky rollout', *Frontiers in Nutrition*, March 2021.

24 'Can estrogen protect against coronavirus? Here are the latest results from the Covid Symptom Study', Covid Symptom Study, May 2021.

25 Seeland, U., Coluzzi, F., Simmaco, M., et al., 'Evidence for treatment with oestradiol for women with SARS-CoV-2 infection', *BMC Medicine*, 18(369).

26 Newson, L. 'Female hormones and Covid-19', Newsonhealth.co.uk, December 2020.

27 'Long-term effects of coronavirus (long COVID)', nhs.uk, July 2021.

28 Longfellow, H. W., 'There was a little girl', 1883.

29 Newson, L., 'Progesterone Intolerance' PDF, menopausedoctor.co.uk, 2020.

30 WHI writers group, 'Risks and benefits of estrogen plus progestins in healthy post-menopausal women', *JAMA*, 2002, 288(3): 321–333.

31 Briden, L. 'The crucial difference between progesterone and progestins', larabriden.com, August 2020.

32 Lieberman, A. and Curtis, L., 'In defense of progesterone: a review of the literature', *Alternative Therapies in Health and Medicine*, 2017, 23(6).

33 Brown-Séquard, C.-E., 'The effects produced on man by subcutaneous injections of a liquid obtained from the testicales of animals', *The Lancet*, July 1889: 105–7.

34 Scott, A. and Newson, L., 'Should we be prescribing testosterone to perimenopausal and menopausal women? A guide to prescribing testosterone for women in primary care', *British Journal of General Practice*, 2020, 70(693): 203–4.

35 Dart, D. A., Waxman, J., Aboagye, E. O., et al., 'Visualising androgen receptor activity in male and female mice', *PLoS ONE*, 2013, 8(8): e71694.

36 'New survey highlights impact of the menopause on every aspect of women's lives in the UK', womens-health-concern.org, October 2017.

37 Marsh, S., 'Viagra prescriptions on NHS triple in 10 years as stigma fades', *Guardian*, August 2017.

38 Fine, C., *Testosterone Rex: Unmaking the Myths of Our Gendered Minds* (Icon Books, 2017).

39 Steinke, D., *Flash Count Diary: Menopause and the Vindication of Natural Life* (Picador, 2019), p.89.

40 Luche, G. D., Boggs, A. S. P., Kucklick, J. R., et al., 'Androstenedione and testosterone but not progesterone are potential biomarkers of

pregnancy in humpback whales (*Megaptera novaeanglia*) approaching parturition', *Scientific Reports*, 2020, 10(2954).
41 Vegunta, S., Kling, J. M. and Kapoor, E., 'Androgen therapy in women', *Journal of Women's Health*, 2020; 29(1): 57–64.
42 Kenny, A. M., Fabregas, G., Song, C., et al., 'Effects of testosterone on behavior, depression, and cognitive function in older men with mild cognitive loss', *Journals of Gerontology*, 2004, Series A, 59(1): M75–78.
43 Davis, S. R., Jane, F., Robinson, P. J., et al., 'Transdermal testosterone improves verbal learning and memory in postmenopausal women not on oestrogen therapy', *Clinical Endocrinology*, 2014, 81(4): 621–8.

CHAPTER 4: THE MENOPAUSE AT WORK

1 Carpenter, J. S., Sheng, Y., Elomba, C. D., et al., 'A systematic review of palpitations prevalence by menopausal status', *Current Obstetrics and Gynecology Reports*, 2021, 10: 7–13.
2 Channel 4/Fawcett Society Menopause and the Workplace Survey, 2022, fawcettsociety.org.uk/menopauseandtheworkplace
3 'Driving the change: menopause and the workplace', circlein.com, 2021.
4 'The menopause: a workplace issue', tuc.org.uk/Wales, June 2017.
5 'New survey highlights impact of the menopause on every aspect of women's lives in the UK', womens-health-concern.org, October 2017.
6 Burden, L., 'Many women exit workforce for a little-talked about reason', bloomberg.com, June 2021.
7 Faragher, J., 'Third of nurses plan to quite NHS in "emerging crisis"', personneltoday.com, September 2020.
8 'BMS, RCOG, RCGP, FSRH, FOM and FPH position Statement in response to the BMA report "Challenging the culture on menopause for doctors"', menopausematters.co.uk, August 2020.
9 Bansal, R. and Aggarwal, N., 'Menopausal hot flashes: a concise review', *Journal of Mid-Life Health*, 2019, 10(1): 6–13.
10 Schaffer, R., 'Hot flashes associated with altered brain function during memory tests', healio.com, January 2020.
11 Maki, P., Drogos, L. L., Rubin, L. H., et al., 'Objective hot flashes are negatively related to verbal memory performance in midlife women', *Menopause*, 2008, 15(5): 848–56.
12 Lucas, R. A. I., Ganio, M. S., Pearson, J., et al., 'Brain blood flow

and cardiovascular reponses to hot flashes in postmenopausal women', *Menopause*, 2013, 20(3): 299–304.
13 Abitbol, J. and Abitbol, B., 'The voice and the menopause: the twilight of the divas', *Contraception, Fertilité, Sexualité*, 1998, 26(9): 649–55.
14 Del Rey, J., 'Amazon tells Sanders and Warren that warehouse workers can pee whenever they want', vox.com, February 2020.
15 Wells, J., 'CIPD launches Flex From 1st campaign,' CIPD.co.uk, February 2021.
16 talkingmenopause.co.uk.
17 'Case No: S/4104575/2017', Employment Tribunals (Scotland), 2018.
18 'Menopause in the workplace: helpful resources', henpicked.net.
19 Channel 4/Fawcett Society Menopause and the Workplace Survey, 2022, fawcettsociety.org.uk/menopauseandtheworkplace
20 'The menopause: a workplace issue', op. cit.
21 Papadatou, A., 'Menopause costs UK economy 14 million working days per year', hrreview.co.uk, April 2019.
22 'Menopause transition: effects on women's economic participation', gov.uk, July 2017.
23 Ibid.
24 Isaac, A., 'Bank of England deputy warns UK economy entering "menopausal" phase', *The Telegraph*, May 2018.
25 Beard, M., 'Mary Beard: A Don's Life: The menopausal economy', *Times Literary Supplement*.
26 'The menopause: a workplace issue', op. cit.
27 Vincent, A., 'Cannes red carpet: women can only go if they wear heels', *The Telegraph*, May 2015.
28 'The MacTaggart Lecture: Dorothy Byrne – Edinburgh TV Festival 2019', *Edinburgh Television Festival*, YouTube, August 2019.

CHAPTER 5: VAGINA AND SEX

1 Theobald, S., *Sex Drive: On the Road to a Pleasure Revolution* (Unbound, 2018).
2 Dodson, B., *Sex for One: The Joy of Selfloving* (Random House, 1987).
3 'New survey highlights impact of the menopause on every aspect of women's lives in the UK', womens-health-concern.org, October 2017.
4 Hambach, A., Evers, S., Summ, O., et al., 'The impact of sexual

activity on idiopathic headaches: an observational study', *Cephalalgia*, 2013, 33(6): 384–9.
5 Theobald, S., *Sex Drive*, op. cit., p.212.
6 Gil, N., '*The Vagina Monologues* is 20 years old but it's more relevant than ever', refinery29.com, September 2018.
7 'Hormone replacement therapy: types', nhs.uk, September 2019.
8 'Menopause and cancer', newsonhealth.co.uk.
9 Thompson, D., 'HRT might help older women ward off recurrent UTIs', consumer.healthday.com, July 2020.
10 'Hormone replacement therapy: types', op. cit.
11 'Drugs and supplements: estrogen (vaginal route): side effects', mayoclinic.org, August 2021.
12 Manson, J. E., Goldstein, S. R., Kagan, R., et al, 'Why the product labeling for low-dose vaginal estrogen should be changed', *Menopause*, 2014, 21(9): 911–16.
13 ACOG Committee Opinion, 'Postmenopausal estrogen therapy route of administration and risk of venous thromboembolism,' acog.org April 2013.
14 Manson, Goldstein, Kagan et al, op. cit.
15 Hemminki, E. and Sihvo, S., 'Finnish Physicians' opinions of vaginal estriol in self-care', *Maturitas*, 1991, 31: 241–7.
16 vagidonna.fi.
17 Mandel, L., '"Big Mouth" season 3 is on a mission to defeat shame', mic.com, October 2019.
18 Panay, N., Briggs, P. and Kovacs, G. T., *Managing the Menopause* (Cambridge University Press, 2020).
19 Elneil, S., 'FGM and FSD: role of surgery', UCL EGA Institute for Women's Health.
20 Lewis, J., *Me and My Menopausal Vagina* (PAL Books, 2018).
21 Ibid., p.109.
22 Järvstråt, L., Spetz, A.-C., Lindh-Åstrand, L., et al., 'Use of hormone therapy in Swedish women aged 80 years or older', *Menopause*, 2019, 22(3): 275–8.
23 Ratcliffe, J., '"Brokenness and holiness really go together": Darcey Steinke on menopause', longreads.com, June 2019.
24 Jane Simpson, *The Pelvic Floor Bible*, (London, Penguin, 2019).
25 Graville, S., 'The "wild wee" network: why midlife women are taking desperate measures to find a lockdown loo', *The Telepgraph*, June 2020.

26 NICE guidelines, 'Menopause diagnosis and management', nice.org.uk, 2015.
27 D'Souza, C., 'How the menopause can make you have an affair: It's one symptom women *don't* expect. But hormone turmoil can drive middle-aged women into the arms of a toyboy', dailymail.co.uk, April 2016.
28 Graville, S., 'Menopause & Me': Christ D'Souza', mpoweredwomen.net, June 2019.
29 'Perimenopause and "sex surge"', mumnset.com, January 2018.
30 Harris, C. (ed.), *M-Boldened: Menopause Conversations We All Need To Have* (Flint Books, 2020), p.112.
31 Ibid., p.118.
32 Richardson, D. and McGeever, J., *Tantric Sex and the Menopause* (Destiny Books, 2018).
33 Pelling, R., 'Fastest way to spice up book club! Blame it on Bridgerton, but the bonkbuster is back. Rowan Pelling rates the raunchiest spring tomes – all written by women', dailymail.co.uk, March 2021.
34 omgyes.com.
35 jodivine.com.

CHAPTER 6: EARLY AND LATE MENOPAUSE

1 'Premature ovarian insufficency', newsonhealth.co.uk.
2 daisynetwork.org.
3 Santoro, N., 'The SWAN song: study of women's health across the nation's recurring themes', *Obstet Gynecol Clin North Am*, 2011 38(3): 417–423.
4 Geronimus, A. T., Hicken, M., Keene, D., et al., '"Weathering" and age patterns of allostatic load scores among Blacks and whites in the United States', *American Journal of Public Health*, 2006, 95(5): 826–33.
5 Geronimus, A. T., Hicken, M. T., Pearson, J. A., et al., 'Do US black women experience stress-related accelerated biological aging? A novel theory and first population-based test of black–white differences in telomere length', *Human Nature*, 2020, 21(1): 19–38.
6 'The British Menopause Society consensus statement on the treatment of premature ovarian insufficiency', thebms.org.uk, 2017.
7 Helen Kemp (ed.), *Surgical Menopause – Not Your Typical Menopause*, lulu.com, GB, 2021, p.7.

8 'The British Menopause Society consensus statement on the treatment of premature ovarian insufficiency', thebms.org.uk, 2017.
9 Georgakis, M. K., Beskou-Kontou, T., Theodoridis, I., et al., 'Surgical menopause in association with cognitive function and risk of dementia: a systematic review and meta-analysis', *Psychoneuroendocrinology*, 2019, 106: 9–19.
10 dianedanzebrink.com.
11 Danzebrink, D., 'Ignorance about menopause is destroying lives – and it's not only women who suffer', *Guardian*, January 2020.
12 Mukhopadhaya, N. and Manyonda, I., 'The hysterectomy story in the United Kingdom', *Journal of Mid-Life Health*, 2013, 4(1): 40–41.
13 Woodward, Z., 'Hysterectomy your questions answered', bmihealth-care.co.uk.
14 Shekhar, C., Paswan, B. and Singh, A., 'Prevalence, sociodemographic determinants and self-reported reasons for hysterectomy in India', *Reproductive Health*, 2019, 16(118).
15 Manson, J., Aragaki, A. K., Bassuk, S. S., et al., 'Menopausal estrogen-alone therapy and health outcomes in women with and without bilateral oophorectomy: a randomized trial', *Annals of Internal Medicine*, 2019, 171(6): 406–14.
16 'Premature ovarian insufficiency', womens-health-concern.org, April 2017.
17 Hamilton, J., 'Early menopausal women could have function restored', bionews.org.uk, April 2021.
18 "Experimental treatment offers hope of fertility to early menopausal women', sciencedaily.com, March 2021.
19 Davies, M., 'Ovarian tissue grafts to combat the menopause', bionews.org.uk, August 2019.
20 Vikström, J., Spetz Holm, A-C., Sydsjö, G., et al., 'Hot flushes still occur in a population of 85-year-old women', *Climacteric*, 2013, 16(3): 453–9.
21 Fluker, M. R., 'HRT in older women: is it ever too late?' *British Columbia Medical Journal*, 2001, 43(9): 517–21.

CHAPTER 7: ALTERNATIVE REMEDIES

1 Stewart, M., 'Are you suffering from Menopause Face? That's how one top expert describes the ravages hormones can wreak in midlife.

Here she reveals how you can turn back time without HRT or Botox', dailymail.co.uk, January 2021.
2 Stewart, M., *Manage Your Menopause Naturally* (New World Library, 2021).
3 North American Menopause Society, 'Obesity can lead to more severe hot flashes and other menopause symptoms', *Science News*, May 2017.
4 'Why alcohol affects women more in menopause', endocrineweb.com, May 2020
5 Mishra N., Mishra V., and Devanshi N., 'Exercise beyond midlife: dos and don'ts', J Midlife Health, July 2011 2(2): 51–56.
6 'Herbal medicines for menopausal symptoms', *Drug and Therapeutics Bulletin*, 2009, 47(1).
7 'Boots Menolieve black cohosh root extract 6.5mg – 30 tablets', boots.com.
8 'Holland & Barrett MenoCool black cohosh 60 tablets', hollandandbarrett.com.
9 'Black cohosh', LiverTox, November 2020.
10 'Black cohosh: fact sheet for health professionals', National Institutes of Health, June 2020.
11 'Black cohosh', LiverTox, op. cit.
12 Chen, L-R., Ko, N-Y. and Chen, K-H., 'Isoflavone supplements for menopausal women: a systematic review', *Nutrients*, 2019, 11(11): 2649.
13 Arnarson, A., '8 surprising health benefits of edamame', healthline.com, February 2017.
14 Neal, D. B., Kahleova, H., Holtz, D. N., 'The women's study for the alleviation of vasomotor symptoms (WAVS)', *Menopause*, July 2021.
15 Nagata, C., Takatsuka, N., Kawakami, N., et al., 'Soy product intake and hot flashes in Japanese women: results from a community-based prospective study', *American Journal of Epidemiology*, 2001, 153(8): 790–3.
16 Rice, S. and Whitehead, S. A., 'Phytoestrogens and breast cancer – promoter or protectors?', *Endocrine-Related Cancer*, 2006, 13(4): 995–1015.
17 Florsheim, L., 'Is the menopause product boom finally here?' *Wall Street Journal Magazine*, August 2020.
18 Ibid.
19 Grinspoon, P., 'Cannabidiol (CBD) – what we know and what we don't, Harvard Health Publishing, April 2020.
20 Shannon, S., Lewis, N., Lee, H., et al., 'Cannabidiol in anxiety and sleep: a large case series', *Permanente Journal*, 2019, 23.

21 Carcieri, C., Tomasello, C., Simiele, M., et al, 'Cannabinoids concentration variability in cannabis olive oil galenic preparations', *Journal of Pharmacy and Pharmacology*, 2018, 70(1): 143–9.

22 'CBD and menopause – help us investigate', satipharm.com.

23 Miller S. et al, 'A systematic review of cannibidiol dosing in clinical populations', Br J Clin Pharmacol, Sept 2019 85(9): 1888–1900.

24 Brewer, S., *CBD: The Essential Guide to Health and Wellness* (Simon and Schuster, 2020).

25 'Cannabis use for menopause symptom management', menopause.org, September 2020.

26 Ibid.

27 Velez, A., 'Why alcohol affects women more in menopause', endocrineweb.com, May 2020.

28 Candy, L. and Halpin, T., 'Stronger: body boosters and booze limiters', *Postcards from Midlife with Lorraine and Trish*, January 2021.

29 'Can a woman have an orgasm after menopause?' ladycare-uk.com, August 2020.

30 'ASA Ruling on LadyCafe Lifetime Ltd', ASA.org.uk, June 2019.

31 'LadyCare menopause magnet: what is it and does it work?' gransnet.com.

32 Martins, V., 'Give your workplace (and yourself) an energy boost in 10 steps', marionglucklinic.com.

33 Valenti, L., 'Now Gwyneth Paltrow and Goop want to "rebrand" menopause', *Vogue*, November 2018.

34 Earle, L., *The Good Menopause Guide* (Orion, 2018).

35 *The Truth About HRT*, lizearlewellbeing.com.

36 North American Menopause Society, 'Treatment of menopause-associated vasomotor symptoms: position statement of the North American Menopause Society', *Menopause*, 2004, 11(1): 11–33.

37 Aschwanden, C., 'Hormone therapy, long shunned for a possible breast cancer link, is now seen as a short-term treatment for menopause symptoms', *Washington Post*, February 2020.

38 'Cognitive behaviour therapy for menopausal symptoms', womens-health-concern.org.

39 5rhythms.com.

40 Tipton, M. J., Collier, N., Massey, H., et al., 'Cold water immersion: kill or cure?' *Experimental Physiology*, 2017, 102(11): 1335–55.

41 Glenny H.,'Cold water swimming: why an icy dip is good for your mental and physical health', sciencefocus.com, July 2020.

42 Knechtle B. et al, 'Cold water swimming – benefits and risks: a narrative review', Int J Environ Res Public Health, Dec 2020 17(23): 8984.
43 Somerfield, H., 'The role of the cold shock protein, RBM3, in cooling synaptic structural plasticity and neuroprotection', repository.cam.ac.uk, 2019.
44 Rowlatt, J., 'Could cold water hold a clue to a dementia cure?', bbc.co.uk/news, October 2020.
45 Buijze, G. A., Sierevelt, I. N., van der Heijden, B. C. J. M., et al., 'The effect of cold showering on health and work: a randomized controlled trial', *PLOS ONE*, 11(9): e0161749.

CHAPTER 8: WHY IS IT SO HARD TO GET HRT?

1 'HRT: Benefits and risks', womens-health-concern.org, November 2020.
2 Renoux, C., Dell'Aniello, S., Garbe, E., et al., 'Transdermal and oral hormone replacement therapy and the risk of stroke: a nested case-control study', bmj.com, 2010.
3 Mueck, A. O., 'Postmenopausal hormone replacement therapy and cardiovascular disease: the value of transdermal oestradiol and micronized progesterone', *Climacteric*, April 2012.
4 Abdi, F., Mobedi, H., Bayat, F., et al., 'The effects of transdermal estrogen delivery on bone mineral density in postmenopausal women: a meta-analysis', *Iranian Journal of Pharmaceutical Research*, 2017, 16(1): 380–89.
5 Botteri, E, Støer, N. C., Sakshaug, S. et al., 'Menopausal hormone therapy and colorectal cancer: a linkage between nationwide registries in Norway', bmjopen.bjm.com, 2017, 7: e017639.
6 Mauvais-Jarvis, F., Manson, J. E., Stevenson, J. C., et al., 'Menopausal hormone therapy and type 2 diabetes prevention: evidence, mechanisms, and clinical implications', *Endocrine Reviews*, 2017, 38(3): 173–88.
7 Roman-Blas, J. A., Castañeda, S., Largo, R., et al., 'Osteoarthritis associated with estrogen deficiency', *Arthritis Research and Therapy*, 2009, 11(5): 241.
8 Tan, M., He, F. J. and MacGregor, G. A., 'Obesity and covid-19: the role of the food industry', bmj.com, 2020, 369.
9 Papadakis, G. E., Hans, D., Gonzalez Rodriguez, E., et al., 'Menopausal hormone therapy is associated with reduced total

and visceral adiposity: the OsteoLaus Cohort', *Journal of Clinical Endocrinology & Metabolism*, 2018, 103(5): 1948–57.

10 Cowley, G., 'The end of the age of estrogen', newsweek.com, July 2002.

11 'HRT: the history', womens-health-concern.org, November 2020.

12 Ibid.

13 Brown, S., 'Shock, terror and controversy: how the media reacted to the Women's Health Initiative', *Climacteric*, 2012, 15(3): 275–80.

14 Rossouw, J. E., Anderson, G. L., Prentice, R. L., et al., 'Risks and benefits of estrogen plus progestin in healthy postmenopausal women: principal results from the Women's Health Initiative randomized controlled trial', *Journal of the American Medical Association*, 2002, 288(3): 321–33.

15 Shapiro, S., Farmer, R. D. T., Mueck, A. O., 'Does hormone replacement therapy cause breast cancer? An application of causal principles to three studies: part 2. The Women's Health Initiative: estrogen plus progestogen', *Journal of Family Planning and Reproductive Health Care*, 2011, 37(3):165–72.

16 Cagnacci, A. and Venier, M., 'The controversial history of hormone replacement therapy', *Medicina*, 2009, 55(9): 602.

17 Panay, N., 'Does hormone replacement therapy cause breast cancer? Commentary on Shapiro et al. papers, Parts 1–5', *Journal of Family Planning and Reproductive Health Care*, 2013, 39: 72–4.

18 Simon, J. A., 'What if the Women's Health Initiative had used transdermal oestradiol and oral progesterone instead?', *Menopause*, 2014, 21(7): 769–83.

19 Trabert, B., Sherman, M. E., Kannan, N., et al., 'Progesterone and breast cancer', *Endocrine Reviews*, 2020, 41(2): 320–44.

20 Rossouw, J. E., Anderson, G. L., Prentice, R. L., et al., 'Risks and benefits of estrogen plus progestin in healthy postmenopausal women', op. cit.

21 Collaborative Group on Hormonal Factors in Breast Cancer, 'Type and timing of menopausal hormone therapy and breast cancer risk: individual participant meta-analysis of the worldwide epidemiological evidence', *The Lancet*, 2019, 394(10204): 1159–68.

22 'The Million Women Study', millionwomenstudy.org

23 Stevenson, J. C. and Farmer, R. D. T., 'HRT and breast cancer: a million women ride again', *Climacteric*, 2020, 23(3): 226–8.

24 Hamoda, H., Panay, N., Pedder, H., et al., 'The British Menopause Society and Women's Health Concern 2020 recommendations

on hormone replacement therapy in menopausal women', *Post Reproductive Health*, 2020, 26(4): 181–209.

25 'BMS, IMS, EMAS, RCOG and AMS Joint Statement', thebms.org.uk, August 2020.

26 'Progestogen and progesterone regimens in HRT: information for patients', Chelsea & Westminster Hospital.

27 Fournier, A., Berrino, F. and Clavel-Chapelon, F., 'Unequal risks for breast cancer associated with different hormone replacement therapies: results from the E3N cohort study', *Breast Cancer Research and Treatment*, 2008, 107(1): 103–111.

28 Ibid.

29 Stevenson, J. C. and Farmer, R. D. T., 'HRT and breast cancer: a million women ride again', op. cit.

30 Hamoda, H., Panay, N., Arya, R., et al., 'The British Menopause Society and Women's Health Concern 2016 recommendations on hormone replacement therapy in menopausal women', *Post Reproductive Health*, 2016.

31 Clark, K. and Westberg, S. M., 'Benefits of levonorgestrel intrauterine device use vs. oral or transdermal progesterone for menopausal women using estrogen containing hormone therapy', *Innovations in Pharmacy*, 2019, 10(3).

32 Hamoda, H., Panay, N., Arya, H., et al., 'The British Menopause Society and Women's Health Concern 2016 recommendations on hormone replacement therapy in menopausal women', op. cit.

33 Stute, P., Wildt, L. and Neulen, J., 'The impact of micronized progesterone on breast cancer risk: a systematic review', *Climacteric*, 2018, 21(2): 111–122.

34 Cordina-Duverger, E., Truong, T., Anger, A., et al., 'Risk of breast cancer by type of menopausal hormone therapy: a case-control study among post-menopausal women in France', *PLoS ONE*, 2013, 8(11): e78016.

35 Éspie, M., Daures, J.-P., Chevallier, T., et al., 'Breast cancer incidence and hormone replacement therapy: results from the MISSION study, prospective phase', *Gynecological Endocrinology*, 2007, 23(7): 391–7.

36 Collaborative Group on Hormonal Factors in Breast Cancer, 'Type and timing of menopausal hormone therapy and breast cancer risk: individual participant meta-analysis of the worldwide epidemiological evidence', op. cit.

37 Lieberman, A. and Curtis, L., 'In defense of progesterone: a review of the literature', *Alternative Therapies in Health and Medicine*, 2017, 23(6).

38 Stanczyk, F. Z., Hapgood, J. P., Winer, S., et al., 'Progestogens used in postmenopausal hormone therapy: differences in their pharmalogical properties, intracellular actions, and clinical effects', *Endocrine Reviews*, 2013, 34(2): 171–208.

39 Fitzpatrick, L. A., Pace, C. and Wiita, B., 'Comparison of regimens containing oral micronized progesterone or medroxyprogesterone acetate on quality of life in menopausal women: a cross-sectional survey', *Journal of Women's Health and Gender-Based Medicine*, 2000, 9(4): 381–7.

40 'Costing report: Menopause: Diagnosis and Management – Implementing the NICE Guideline on the Menopause (NG23)', nice.org.uk, November 2013.

41 Karim, R., Dell, R. M., Green, D. F., et al., 'Hip fracture in postmenopausal women after cessation of hormone therapy: results from a prospective study in a large health management organization', *Menopause*, 2011, 18(11); 1172–7.

42 Maclaran, K. and Stevenson, J. C., 'Primary prevention of cardiovascular disease with HRT', *Women's Health*, 2012, 8(1): 63–74.

43 Hamoda, H., Panay, N., Arya, R., et al., 'The British Menopause Society and Women's Health Concern 2016 recommendations on hormone replacement therapy in menopausal women', op. cit.

44 'My morning routine!! (Pssst includes how I apply my HRT)', *Davina McCall*, YouTube, April 2021.

45 'Ongoing shortages of HRT and contraceptives remain unacceptable and continue to harm women, say professional bodies', rcog.org.uk, February 2020.

46 'FRSH press release: Ongoing shortages of HRT and contraceptives remain unacceptable and continue to harm women, say professional bodies', fsrh.org, February 2020.

47 Writing Group of the Women's Health Initiative Investigators, 'Risks and benefits of estrogen plus progestin in health post-menopausal women: principal results from the Women's Health Initiative Randomized Controlled Trial', *Journal of the American Medical Association*, 2002, 288(3): 321–33.

48 Bezwada, P., Shaikh, A. and Misra, D., 'The effect of transdermal estrogen patch use on cardiovascular outcomes: a systematic review', *Journal of Women's Health*, 2017, 26(12): 1319–25.

49 Abdi, F., Mobedi, H., Bayat, F., et al., 'The effects of transdermal estrogen delivery on bone mineral density in postmenopausal women: a meta-analysis', *Iranian Journal of Pharmaceutical Research*, 2017, 16(1): 380–9.

50 'Hormone Repacement Therapy (HRT)', theros.org.uk, 2021.

51 Gera, R., Tayeh, S., El-Hage Chehade, H., et al., 'Does transdermal testosterone increase the risk of developing breast cancer? A systematic review', *Anticancer Research*, 2018, 38(12): 6615–20.

52 'Study suggests testosterone may help ease menopausal symptoms without increasing breast cancer risk', breastcancer.org, 2013.

53 Newson, L. and Mair, R., 'Results from the BJFM menopause survey', *British Journal of Family Medicine*, 2018, 6(1).

54 'Menopause: diagnosis and management: NICE guideline [N23]', nice.org.uk, November 2015.

55 Cordina-Duverger, E., Truong, T., Anger, A., et al., 'Risk of breast cancer by type of menopausal hormone therapy: a case-control study among post-menopausal women in France', op. cit.

56 'The Great Testosterone Postcode Lottery – Template Letter for Your CCG', menopausesupport.co.uk.

57 'Testosterone replacement in menopause', thebms.org.uk.

58 'Testosterone patches for female sexual dysfunction', *Drug and Therapeutics Bulletin*, 2009, 47: 30–34.

59 Newon, L. 'Joining the dots with perimenopause symptoms', nursinginpractice.com, July 2021.

60 Hillman, S., Shantikumar, S., Ridha, Al, et al., 'Socioeconomic status and HRT prescribing: a study of practice-level data in England', *British Journal of General Practice*, 2020, 70(700): e772–7.

61 Martin, D. M., Kukumani, S., Martin, M., et al., 'Learning disabilities and the menopause', *Journal of the British Menopause Society*, 2003, 9(1): 22–6.

62 Millard, L. and McCarthy, M., *Supporting Women with Learning Disabilities Through the Menopause: A Resource Pack,* Second edition (Pavilion, 2017).

63 'Understanding the risks of breast cancer', womens-health-concern.org, 2015.

64 Stute, P., Wildt, L. and Neulen, J., 'The impact of micronized progesterone on breast cancer risk: a systematic review', op. cit.

65 Abenhaim et al, 'Menopausal Hormone Therapy Formulation and Breast Cancer Risk', *Obstet Gynecol*, 2022, June 1;139(6): 1103-1110.

66 Éspie, M., Daures, J.-P., Chevallier, T., et al., 'Breast cancer incidence

and hormone replacement therapy: results from the MISSION study, prospective phase', *Gynecological Endocrinology*, 2007, 23(7): 391–7.
67 'WHI randomized study long term follow up results – December 2019: HRT and breast cancer', thebms.org.uk, 2019.
68 Chlebowski, R. T., Anderson, G. L. and Aragaki, A. K., 'Association of menopausal hormone therapy with breast cancer incidence and mortality during long-term follow-up of the Women's Health Initiative Randomized Clinical Trials', *Journal of the American Medical Association*, 2020, 324(4): 369–80.
69 Paganini-Hill, A., Corrada, M. M. and Kawas, C. H., 'Increased longevity in older users of postmenopausal oestrogen therapy: the Leisure World Cohort Study', *Menopause*, 2018, 25(11): 1256–61.
70 Cordina-Duverger, E., Truong, T., Anger, A., et al., 'Risk of breast cancer by type of menopausal hormone therapy: a case-control study among post-menopausal women in France', op. cit.
71 'Hormone replacement therapy - number of U.S. women using at least one drug 2001-2008', statista.com, November 2011.
72 Sarrel P., Njike V., Vinante V. , Katz D., 'The Mortality Toll of Estrogen Avoidance: An Analysis of Excess Deaths Among Hysterectomized Women Aged 50 to 59 Years', *Am J Public Health,* 2013, 103(9): 1583–1588.
73 'BMS, IMS, EMAS, RCOG and AMS Joint Statement', op. cit.

CHAPTER 9: THE RISKY BUSINESS OF MENOPAUSE

1 healthandher.com.
2 'Hormone replacement therapy and menopause testing', onlinedoctor.superdrug.com.
3 gennev.com.
4 femalefoundersfund.com.
5 'Search results for HRT: Hormone replacement therapy', nhs.uk.
6 Mirkin, S., 'Evidence on the use of progesterone in menopausal hormone therapy', *Climacteric*, 2018, 1(4): 346–54.
7 londonhormoneclinic.com.
8 marionglucklinic.com.
9 Winterson, J., 'Jeanette Winterson: can you stop the menopause', *Guardian*, April 2014.

10 'Remote HRT prescribing', My Menopause Doctor, YouTube, November 2020.
11 Newson, L. and Mair, R., 'Results from the BJFM menopause survey', *British Journal of Family Medicine*, 2018, 6(1).
12 Kling, J. M., MacLaughlin, K. L., Schnatz, P. F., et al., 'Menopause management knowledge in postgraduate family medicine, internal medicine, and obstetrics and gynecology residents: a cross-sectional survey', *Mayo Clinic Proceedings*, 2019, 94(2): 242–53.
13 'Menopause care for women', newsonhealth.co.uk, 2019.
14 'BMS consensus statement: bioidentical HRT', thebms.org.uk, October 2019.
15 'Hormone replacement therapy: alternatives', nhs.uk, September 2019.
16 'Standards for registered pharmacies', pharmacyregulation.org.
17 'Use our inspection reports to find and compare care services', cqc.org.uk.
18 Thompson, J. J., Ritenbaugh, C. and Nichter, M., 'Why women choose compounded bioidentical hormone therapy: lessons from a qualitative study of menopausal decision-making', *BMC Women's Health*, 2017, 17(97).
19 North American Menopause Society, 'More women using compounded hormones without understanding the risks', sciencedaily.com, February 2015.
20 'Compounding and the FDA: Questions and answers', fda.gov, June 2018.
21 'Statement on improving adverse event reporting of compound drugs to protect patients', fda.gov, September 2019.
22 Jakobson Ramin, C., 'The hormone hoax thousands fall for', *More*, October 2013.
23 Stroumsa, D., Crissman, H. P., Dalton, V., K., et al., 'Insurance coverage and use of hormones among transgender respondants to a national survey', *Annals of Family Medicine*, 2020, 18(6): 528–34.
24 'Lydia Pinkham', wikipedia.org.

CHAPTER 10: THE MENOPAUSE AND BREAST CANCER

1 'Breast cancer (invasive) statistics', cancerresearchuk.org.
2 'How common is breast cancer', cancer.org, May 2021.
3 'Cancer statistics by cancer type', cancerresearchuk.org.
4 'Breast cancer survival statistics', cancerresearchuk.org.

5 'BRCA1 and BRCA2 genes', mskcc.org.
6 Sulik, G., 'Angelina Jolie and the one percent', *Scientific American*, May 2013.
7 'Tools for clinicians', thebms.org.uk.
8 Baum, M., *The History and Mystery of Breast Cancer* (Cambridge Scholars Publishing, 2019).
9 lattelounge.co.uk.
10 'Letrozole', nhs.uk.
11 Mufudza, C., Sorofa, W. and Chiyaka, E. T., 'Assessing the effects of estrogen on the dynamics of breast cancer', *Computational and Mathematical Methods in Medicine*, 2012, 473572.
12 Chlebowski, R. T., Anderson, G. L., Aragaki, K. A., et al., 'Association of menopausal hormone therapy with breast cancer incidence and mortality during long-term follow-up of the Women's Health Initiative randomized clinical trials', *Journal of the American Medical Association*, 2020, 324(4): 369–80.
13 Crist, C., 'Breast cancer survivors face other health risks after treatment', reuters.com, December 2019.
14 'Using vaginal oestrogen not linked to high breast cancer risk', breastcancer.org, August 2017.
15 Newson, L. 'Menopause and cancer', menopausedoctor.co.uk.
16 Bluming, A., 'Hormone replacement therapy (HRT) in women with previously treated breast cancer. Update XI', *Journal of Clinical Oncology*, 23(16 – supplement): 787.
17 Bluming, A. and Tavris, C., *Oestrogen Matters* (Piatkus, 2018), p.168.
18 Ibid., p.192.
19 Holmberg, L., Anderson, H. and HABITS steering and data monitoring committees, 'HABITS (hormone replacement therapy after breast cancer – is it safe?), a randomised comparison: trial stopped', *The Lancet*, 2004, 363(9407):453–5.
20 Fahlén, M., Fornander, T., Johansson, H., et al., 'Hormone replacement therapy after breast cancer: 10 year follow up of the Stockholm randomised trial', *European Journal of Cancer*, 2013, 49(1): 52–9.
21 Early Breast Cancer Trialists' Collaborative Group (EBCTCG), 'Aromatase inhibitors versus tamoxifen in early breast cancer: patient-level meta-analysis of the randomised trials', *The Lancet*, 2015, 386(10001): 1341–52.
22 Southall, J., 'Exercise has "astounding" effect on breast cancer recurrence, mortality', healio.com, May 2017.

23 Playdon M. et al, 'Weight Gain After Breast Cancer Diagnosis and All-Cause Mortality: Systematic Review and Meta-Analysis', *J Natl Cancer Inst* 2015 107(12): djv275.
24 Fenlon, D., Maishman, T., Day, L., et al., 'Effectiveness of nurse-led group CBT for hot flushes and night sweats in women with breast cancer: results of the MENOS4 randomised controlled trial', *Psycho-Oncology*, 2020, 29(10).
25 'Breast cancer survivors face elevated risk of suicide', news.cancerconnect.com, 2018.
26 'A beginners guide to BRCA1 an BRCA2', The Royal Marsden NHS Foundation Trust, 2016.
27 Jolie, A., 'My medical choice', *New York Times*, May 2013.
28 Marsden, J. on behalf of the British Menopause Society, 'British Menopause Society consensus statement: The risks and benefits of HRT before and after a breast cancer diagnosis', *Post Reproductive Health*, 2019, 25(1): 33–7.
29 Obermiller, P. S., Tait, D. L. and Holt, J. T., 'Gene therapy for carcinoma of the breast: therapeutic gene correction strategies', *Breast Cancer Research*, 2000, 2(1): 28–31.
30 'Health & Ancestry Service', 23andme.com.
31 Jones, J., 'Hendrickje Stoffels, Rembrandt (c.1654–60)', *Guardian*, August 2001.
32 'Hendrickje Stoffels', wikipedia.com.

CHAPTER 11: DO HORMONES HELP PREVENT ALZHEIMER'S DISEASE?

1 Sauer, A., 'Why is Alzheimer's more likely in women?' Alzheimers.net, September 2019.
2 '053 the costs of the menopause – Professor Philip Sarrel and Dr Louise Newson', menopausedoctor.co.uk, 23 June 2020.
3 Maki, P., 'Hot flashes associated with altered brain function during memory tests', healio.com, January 2020.
4 Kim, Y. J., Soto, M., Branigan, G. L., et al., 'Association between menopausal hormone therapy and risk of neurodegenerative diseases: implications for precision hormone therapy', *Alzheimer's and Dementia*, 2021, 7(1): e12174.
5 Mosconi, L., *The XX Brain: The Groundbreaking Science Empowering Women to Prevent Dementia* (Allen & Unwin, 2021).

6 'Alzheimer's and women's health: an urgent call', lisamosconi.com.
7 Rettberg, J. R., Yao, J., Brinton, R. D., 'Estrogen: a master regulator of bioenergetics systems in the brain and body', *Frontiers in Neuroendocrinology*, 2014, 35(1): 8–30.
8 Rocca, W. A., Grossardt, B. R., Schuster, L. T., et al., 'Hysterectomy, oophorectomy, estrogen and the risk of dementia', *Neurodegenerative Diseases*, 2012, 10(1–4): 175–8.
9 Mosconi, L., Berti, V., Dyke, J., et al., 'Menopause impacts human brain structure, connectivity, energy metabolism, and amyloid-beta deposition', *Scientific Reports*, 2021, 11(10867).
10 'We need to know how menopause changes women's brains', *New York Times*, July 2021.
11 'Roberta Diaz Brinton, PhD: Women and Alzheimer's Disease', *SOUL Food Salon*, YouTube, October 2017.
12 Robertson, S., 'Oestradiol and the brain', news-medical.net, May 2021.
13 Klosinski, L. P., Yao., J., Yin, F., et al, 'White matter lipids as a ketogenic fuel supply in aging female brain: implications for Alzheimer's disease', *ebiomedicine*, 2015, 2(12): 1888–1904.
14 'The future of dementia is orange,' alzheimersresearchuk.org, 2016.
15 Cintron, D., Lahr, B. D., Bailey, K. R., et al., 'Effects of oral versus transdermal menopausal hormone treatments on self-reported sleep domains and their association with vasomotor symptoms in recently menopausal women enrolled in the Kronos Early Estrogen Prevention Study (KEEPS)', *Menopause*, 2018, 25(2): 145–53.
16 'Sleep and Alzheimer's disease – more evidence on their relationship,' alzdiscovery.org, Feb 2019.
17 Cordone, S., Annarumma, L., Rossini, P. et al, 'Sleep and ß-amyloid deposition in Alzheimer's disease: insights on mechanisms and possible innovative treatments', *Frontiers in Pharmacology*, 2019, 10: 695.
18 'Mediterranean diet may protect against Alzheimer's disease', Weill Cornell Medicine, May 2018.
19 Cording J.' 'Little life hacks to support a healthy female brain,' forbes.com, March 2020.
20 Greenlaw. L, 'The Sea is an Edge and an Ending,' *The Built Moment* (Faber, 2019).
21 Mosconi, L. *The XX Brain*, op. cit., p.129.
22 Ragson, N. L., Geist, G. L, Kenna, H. A., et al., 'Prospective randomized trail to assess effects of continuing hormone therapy on

cerebral function in postmenopausal women at risk from dementia', *PLoS ONE*, 2014, 9(3): e89095.

23 Monstra, M., 'Brain effects of menopausal HT differ for pill, patch delivery', healio.com, October 2020.

24 Kling, J. M., Miller, V. M., Tosakulwong, N., et al., 'Associations of pituitary-ovarian hormones and white matter hyperintensities in recently menopausal women using hormone therapy', *Menopause*, 2020, 27(8): 872–8.

25 Robertson, D., Craig, M., van Amelsvoort, T., et al., 'Effects of estrogen therapy on age-related differences in gray matter concentration', *Climacteric*, 2009, 12(4): 301–9.

26 Kim, Y. J., Soto, M., Branigan, G. L., et al., 'Association between menopausal hormone therapy and risk of neurodegenerative diseases: implications for precision hormone therapy', op. cit.

27 Pham, T. M., Petersen, I., Walters, K., et al., 'Trends in dementia diagnosis rates in UK ethnic groups: analysis of UK primary care data', *Clinical Epidemiology*, 2081, 10: 949–60.

28 Ozuzu Nwaiwu, J., 'Black women's perceptions of menopause and the use of hormone replacement therapy', *Nursing Times*, 2007.

29 Wenshan, Lv., Du, N., Liu, Y., et al., 'Low testosterone level and risk of Alzheimer's disease in the elderly men: a systematic review and meta-analysis', *Molecular Neurobiology*, 2016, 53(4): 2679–84.

30 'Hormones and dementia', alzheimers.org.uk.

31 ' Hormone therapy linked to small Alzheimer's risk increase' and 'Study finds to link between hormone therapy and Alzheimer's risk', alzheimersresearchuk.org.

32 Gates, B., 'Data could hold the key to stopping Alzheimer's', gatesnotes.com, November 2020.

CHAPTER 12: THE ANDROPAUSE, MENOPAUSE AND RELATIONSHIPS

1 Sawalha, N., 'How Nadia's menopause pushed Mark to the edge & how men should deal with hormones'; 'Has HRT (hormone replacement therapy) saved our marriage?!' *How to Stay Married (So Far)*.

2 Casimiro, I. and Cohen, R. N., 'Severe vasomotor symptoms post-oophorectomy despite testosterone therapy in a transgender man: a unique case study, *Journal of the Endocrine Society*, 2019, 3(4): 734–6.

3 Letter from Ernest Hemingway to Maxwell Perkins in Hemingway, E., *Selected Letters, 1917–1961*, ed. Baker, C. (Granada, 1981), p.395.

4 Larsen, L., *Stein and Hemingway: The Story of a Turbulent Friendship* (McFarland and Co., 2011), p77.

5 Ibid., p.96.

6 Hemingway, E., *Selected Letters 1917-1961*, op. cit, p387–8; McAuliffe, M., *Paris on the Brink: The 1930s Paris of Jean Renoir, Salvador Dalí, Simone de Beauvoir, André Gide, Sylvia Beach, Léon Blum, and their Friends* (Roman & Littlefield, 2020), p.120.

7 Larsen, p.49.

8 Ibid., p.123.

9 Foster, J. *Man Alive: The Health Problems Men Face and How to Fix Them* (Piatkus, 2021).

10 British Society for Sexual Medicine, 'British Society for Sexual Medicine guidelines on adult testosterone deficiency, with statements for UK practice', guidelines.co.uk, January 2018.

11 Patterson, D., McInnes, G. T., Webster, J., et al., 'Influence of a single dose of 20mg tadalafil, a phosphodieterase 5 inhibitor, on ambulatory blood pressure in subjects with hypertension', *British Journal of Clinical Pharmacology*, 2006, 62(3): 280–87.

12 'Dataset: Divorces in England and Wales', ons.gov.uk, November 2020.

13 Colas, K., 'Divorce statistics are high at menopause and women are often the instigators', womens-health-concern.org, September 2015.

14 libertychoir.org.

CHAPTER 13: FEMINISM AND THE FUTURE

1 Burney-Scott, O., *The Black Girl's Guide to Surviving Menopause*, Blackgirlsguidetosurvivingmenopause.com.

2 pausitivity.co.uk.

3 'NICEImpact: Falls and fragility fractures', nice.org.uk, July 2018.

4 'Listening to Estrogen', thect.com, December 2018.

5 Salami, M., *Sensuous Knowledge: A Black Feminist Approach for Everyone* (Zed Books, 2020).

6 menopausecafe.net.

7 menopausesupport.co.uk.

8 @drnighatarif, TikTok and Instagram.

9 Millard, L. and McCarthy, M., *Supporting Women with Learning Disabilities Through the Menopause: A Resource Pack,* Second edition (Pavilion, 2017).

INDEX